201 Careers in Nursing

JOYCE J. FITZPATRICK, PhD, MBA, RN, FAAN, FNAP

EMERSON E. EA, DNP, APRN, BC, CEN

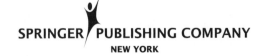

SPRINGER PUBLISHING COMPANY

NEW YORK

Springer Publishing Company, LLC
11 West 42nd Street
New York, NY 10036
www.springerpub.com

Acquisitions Editor: Allan Graubard
Composition: Newgen Imaging

ISBN: 978-0-8261-3382-3
E-book ISBN: 978-0-8261-3383-0

12 13/ 5 4 3 2

The author and the publisher of this Work have made every effort to use sources believed to be reliable to provide information that is accurate and compatible with the standards generally accepted at the time of publication. Because medical science is continually advancing, our knowledge base continues to expand. Therefore, as new information becomes available, changes in procedures become necessary. We recommend that the reader always consult current research and specific institutional policies before performing any clinical procedure. The author and publisher shall not be liable for any special, consequential, or exemplary damages resulting, in whole or in part, from the readers' use of, or reliance on, the information contained in this book. The publisher has no responsibility for the persistence or accuracy of URLs for external or third-party Internet Web sites referred to in this publication and does not guarantee that any content on such Web sites is, or will remain, accurate or appropriate.

Library of Congress Cataloging-in-Publication Data

Fitzpatrick, Joyce J., 1944-
   201 careers in nursing / Joyce J. Fitzpatrick, Emerson E. Ea.
      p. ; cm.
   Two hundred one careers in nursing
   Two hundred and one careers in nursing
   Includes index.
   ISBN 978-0-8261-3382-3 — ISBN 978-0-8261-3383-0 (e-ISBN)
   1. Nursing—Vocational guidance—United States. I. Ea, Emerson E. II. Title. III. Title: Two hundred one careers in nursing. IV. Title: Two hundred and one careers in nursing.
   [DNLM: 1. Career Choice—United States. 2. Nursing—United States. 3. Vocational Guidance—United States. WY 16 AA1]
   RT82.F58 2011
   610.7306'9—dc23   2011022924

Special discounts on bulk quantities of our books are available to corporations, professional associations, pharmaceutical companies, health care organizations, and other qualifying groups.

If you are interested in a custom book, including chapters from more than one of our titles, we can provide that service as well.

For details, please contact:
Special Sales Department, Springer Publishing Company, LLC
11 West 42nd Street, 15th Floor, New York, NY 10036-8002
Phone: 877-687-7476 or 212-431-4370; Fax: 212-941-7842
Email: sales@springerpub.com

Printed in the United States of America by Bang Printing.

■ CONTENTS

Contents

Contents

Contents

Contents

■ INTRODUCTION

We, the authors of this book, are passionate about nursing and the career opportunities within the nursing profession. We have had many opportunities within our own careers to expand our roles, and to contribute to quality patient care, nursing and health care science, and to make the world a better place for patient and their families, for the communities in which we live and work, and importantly, the citizens of the world.

We firmly believe that there is no other career that has as much potential for personal and professional satisfaction. A career in nursing offers opportunities to care for others from infancy to the older adult, from those who need health information to those experiencing a terminal illness. Nurses work with individuals and families at their most vulnerable times of illness and have the most intimate relationships with patients. Nurses are there in time of need. They are in hospitals 24 hours a day, 7 days a week, 365 days a year, monitoring every aspect of patient care. They are in communities, delivering home care to those who are house-bound due to illness or injury, providing health education in schools, in wellness centers, and in medical offices. They are aboard cruise ships and on resorts, and they transport patients, via helicopter or ambulance, when care is necessary at another facility. Nursing is ...listening to the cries of a newborn and the joys of the parents; being with a older woman who has a fractured hip who knows she will no longer be able to live independently; tending to the wounds of those in combat, and understanding how anxious they are to return to their loved ones at the same time they want to serve their country; soothing the pain of the person recovering from surgery, and studying the effects of new treatments for cancer, cardiovascular disease, and many other illnesses. As you will discover in this book, nurses have the choice of a myriad of careers. We have identified the 201 most prominent careers in nursing at this time. We have provided information so that the reader is introduced to opportunities within and across the careers. For example, many nurses combine careers as educators, teaching part time in schools of nursing, and expert clinicians, working clinically as advanced practice nurses in hospitals and health centers. Nurses who hold academic appointments combine their teaching role with that as researcher. Nurses who work in management often combine their administrative work with writing and lecturing.

If you are considering a career in nursing, this book will introduce you to the wide range of career choices. You will be surprised and impressed with the many career choices available. As I have talked with potential students, who have over a period of time realized that a career in nursing might be for them, they have mentioned the stereotypes that are still prevalent in the public view of nursing. Indeed there are strong stereotypes, many of which are dated to years ago when there was little education required of nurses and when much of the work was task oriented and rote rather than requiring the high level clinical judgment and skills needed today.

If you know someone who is considering a career in nursing, this book is a very good overview. Many prospective nurses are not aware of the broad range of opportunities, even though they may have decided on the career choice. I often hear people say that they could never be a nurse as they do not like the "blood and guts" aspect of care. Granted there is some dimension of the educational program that requires the nursing student to experience bloody procedures, there are many career choices where there is no blood. Read about the possibilities in psychiatric or community health nurse, in historical or ethical research, or in executive positions.

If you are a guidance counselor, this book will help you learn more about the profession of nursing. You will be better prepared to advise others about the educational requirements and the competencies necessary for the specific careers.

If you are a nurse and considering a change in your career, this book will help you identify the range of opportunities and the skill sets necessary for each career. You may decide to return to school to gain more education to prepare yourself for the new career, or you may learn more about a particular career by shadowing an expert nurse who is already in that career.

How should you use this book to find a job in nursing? First you should acquaint yourself with the range of possibilities: review the table of contents for the list of career choices in nurses. Next, eliminate some of these options. If you have an interest in older adults look first at the descriptions within geriatric nursing. If you are more interested in caring for children there are a range of careers for pediatric nurses that are described here. The following tips will help you in your search of career or job within nursing:

- Consider the factors that are most important in your life; if you like being with and helping others then a career in nursing could be right for you.
- Ask yourself why you might want to do a particular kind of work; self-assessment is an important part of a career choice.
- Think about nursing as a career, not just a job choice; engage in some long-range planning as well as short term consideration of job opportunities.
- Decide if you have any parameters to rule out, for example, age group.
- Consider the place of employment; some people are petrified of hospitals, yet they might make good community health nurses.
- Select what you might consider the "top 10" careers of interest.
- Read the basic description provided for the careers that might interest you.
- Review the educational requirements for the career; if you have this educational background you are prepared to pursue the career. If you do not have the required educational background but are still interested in the career, decide how you will become prepared. There are many formal college and university programs and continuing education opportunities that are available and many provide flexible schedules for the student or the nurse who has to continue to work full time.
- Review the core competencies that are needed to be successful in the career. If you do not already possess these competencies, decide how you will prepare yourself.
- Develop your resume, highlighting your experiences and competencies that qualify you for the new career.
- Learn as much as you can about the position; access the web sites that are listed for each career in order to obtain more detailed information.
- Ask others what they know about the career; plan to meet someone who is already in that career. Today the internet makes it possible to reach out to others across the globe in order to

obtain information. Schedule a time to meet with or talk with someone who is in the career of your choice. Ideally you also would find an opportunity to "shadow" the person in their place of employment for at least a day.

- Networking with others is an important part of career development; you should take every opportunity to meet others and continue to network with them throughout your career development.
- Consider all opportunities carefully: Many opportunities for career advancement will come your way; consider each opportunity and decide if it fits into your overall career goals.
- Develop an action plan to get you where you want to be in your career; make certain you have carefully considered the time frame that will be necessary for you to achieve your goals.
- Let others know, as many people as possible, that you are interested in a particular career in nursing. There is a strong network of nurses in key positions who could be helpful to you in your career search; do not hesitate to approach others for help.
- Find a mentor who can help you with your continuing professional development over the life of your career.
- Continue to build your skills in your new position and maintain your contacts for future job searches.

What binds these many nursing career opportunities are the values of the profession. Nursing is a caring profession, built on the belief that as humans we are all striving toward health. Nurses have a commitment to help individuals obtain and maintain health through education, therapeutic interventions and evaluations of the care provided. As professionals nurses have a societal responsibility to help others move toward health and wellness.

We believe that the descriptions of each of the careers in this book reflect the core dimensions of nursing, the caring, competence and commitment to excellence and to serving people in their time of need. We are proud to be nurses. Through this book we want to spread the word, not only of the value of our profession, but also of the benefits to individuals who choose a career in nursing.

Joyce J. Fitzpatrick
Emerson E. Ea

■ ABOUT THE AUTHORS

Joyce J. Fitzpatrick, PhD, MBA, RN, FAAN, FNAP, is the Elizabeth Brooks Ford Professor of Nursing, Frances Payne Bolton School of Nursing, Case Western Reserve University (CWRU) in Cleveland, OH, where she was Dean from 1982 through 1997. She holds an adjunct position as Professor in the Department of Geriatrics, Mount Sinai School of Medicine, New York, NY. She earned a BSN at Georgetown University, Washington, DC; an MS in Psychiatric–Mental Health Nursing at The Ohio State University, Columbus, OH; a PhD in Nursing at New York University, New York, NY; and an MBA from CWRU in 1992. In May, 1990, Dr. Fitzpatrick received an honorary doctorate, Doctor of Humane Letters, from her alma mater, Georgetown University. She 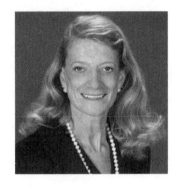 has received numerous honors and awards; she was elected a Fellow in the American Academy of Nursing in 1981, and in 1996 a Fellow in the National Academies of Practice. She has received the *American Journal of Nursing* Book of the Year Award 18 times. In 2002, Dr. Fitzpatrick received the American Nurses Foundation Distinguished Contribution to Nursing Science Award for her sustained commitment and contributions to the development of the discipline. In 2003, she received the STTI Lucie Kelly Mentor Award, and in 2005, she received the STTI Founders Award for Leadership. From 2007 to 2008 she served as a Fulbright Scholar at University College Cork, Cork, Ireland.

Dr. Fitzpatrick is widely published in nursing and health care literature having over 300 publications. She served as coeditor of the *Annual Review of Nursing Research* series, volumes 1 through 26; she currently edits the journals *Applied Nursing Research, Archives in Psychiatric Nursing*, and *Nursing Education Perspectives*, the official journal of the National League for Nursing. Dr. Fitzpatrick was coauthor of the book, *101 Careers in Nursing*, published by Springer Publishing. Her recent books published by Springer Publishing Company include *Giving through Teaching: How Nurse Educators* Are Changing the World, published in June 2010 and *Problem Solving for Better Health: A Global Perspective* published in November 2010.

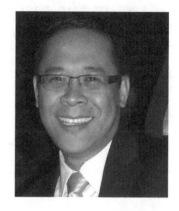

Emerson E. Ea, DNP, APRN, BC, CEN, is Clinical Assistant Professor and Senior Clinical Faculty Associate, Hartford Institute for Geriatric Nursing at New York University College of Nursing. He is a Board Certified Adult Nurse Practitioner and Medical–Surgical Nurse by the American Nurses Credentialing Center and is an Emergency Room Nurse certified by the Board of Certification for Emergency Nursing. He obtained his Bachelor of Science in Nursing from University of St. La Salle, Bacolod City, Philippines, his Master's of Science specializing in Adult Health from Long Island University, Brooklyn Campus, Brooklyn, NY, and his Doctor of Nursing Practice with a focus on Educational Leadership at Case Western Reserve University, Cleveland, OH. He is also a recipient of a scholarship from Thomas Edison State College, Trenton, NJ, where he completed a Certificate in Distance Learning. His scholarship interests include acculturation among immigrant nurses especially Filipino Registered Nurses, cardiovascular health among Filipino Americans, and geriatric nursing.

201 Careers in Nursing

1 ■ ACUPUNCTURIST NURSE

BASIC DESCRIPTION
An acupuncturist nurse is a holistic practitioner based on Traditional Chinese Medicine's concept of integrative health. The acupuncturist nurse uses needles, heat or pressure to promote wellness, health, and balance. They are employed by ambulatory centers and holistic care centers.

EDUCATIONAL REQUIREMENTS
Registered Nurse is preferred; certification could be obtained from the National Certification Commission for Acupuncture and Oriental Medicine.

CORE COMPETENCIES/SKILLS NEEDED
Additional education and training in holistic medicine are required

- Knowledge of anatomy and Centers for Disease Control infection control standards
- Excellent communication and interpersonal skills

RELATED WEB SITES AND PROFESSIONAL ORGANIZATIONS
- National Certification Commission for Acupuncture and Oriental Medicine (www.nccaom.org)
- The American Association of Acupuncture and Oriental Medicine (www.aaaomonline.org)

2 ■ ACUTE CARE NURSE PRACTITIONER

BASIC DESCRIPTION

Acute care nurse practitioners are advanced practice nurses who specialize in providing care for acutely ill patients in a variety of settings. The environment in which acute care nurse practitioners function is very intense and dramatic. Some of the characteristics of an acute care nurse practitioner's work include coordinating patient care, assessing the patient's health history, ordering diagnostic tests, performing therapeutic procedures, and prescribing medications. Possibilities to work exist in:

- Emergency rooms
- Operating rooms
- Critical care units
- Transplant units

EDUCATIONAL REQUIREMENTS

Master of Science in Nursing with advanced practice certification as an Acute Care Nurse Practitioner is required. Graduate programs are generally 2 years in length. The number of schools that offer this specialty is limited; therefore, entry into these programs is competitive. Certification is available from the American Nurses Credentialing Center or the American Association of Critical Care Nurses.

CORE COMPETENCIES/SKILLS NEEDED

- Technical competency involving use of complex and computerized equipment
- Regulating ventilators
- Hemodynamic monitoring
- Obtaining blood samples from central IV lines
- Interpersonal competency dealing with patients and their families in life-threatening situations

- Ability to work with interdisciplinary teams
- Extensive experience and expertise in assessing and managing acutely ill patients

RELATED WEB SITES AND PROFESSIONAL ORGANIZATIONS

- American Association of Nurse Practitioners (www.aanp.org)
- Nurse Practitioner Support Services (www.nurse.net)
- Cost and Quality: The Emergence of the Acute Care Nurse Practitioner (www.cost-quality.com)
- Nurse Practitioner Associates for Continuing Education (www.npace.org)
- American Nurses Association Credentialing Center (www.nursecredentialing.org)
- American Association of Critical Care Nurses (www.aacn.org)

3 ■ ADDICTIONS COUNSELOR

BASIC DESCRIPTION

Nurses who are addictions counselors work in organizations that specialize in helping clients overcome addictive disorders. Treatment programs exist in all regions of the country. Chemical dependency is a major health problem, and nurses work with clients to help them learn more effective ways of coping.

EDUCATIONAL REQUIREMENTS

Bachelor of Science in Nursing is preferred with certification as a Certified Addictions Registered Nurse (CARN). Three years' experience as an RN is necessary for CARN certification. Within the 5 years prior to the application for certification, a minimum of 4,000 hours (2 years) of nursing experience related to addictions is required. There is also an advanced practice certification that requires the Master of Science in Nursing.

CORE COMPETENCIES/SKILLS NEEDED
- Excellent interpersonal and counseling skills
- Good interviewing techniques
- Strong assessment skills
- Counseling ability
- Compassion and empathy
- Interest in mental health
- Ability to work in interdisciplinary teams

RELATED WEB SITES AND PROFESSIONAL ORGANIZATIONS
- International Nurses Society on Addictions (www.intnsa.org)
- American Nurses Association Peer Assistance Program (www.ana.org)

4 ■ ADMINISTRATOR/MANAGER

BASIC DESCRIPTION
Nurse administrators and executive directors are needed in numerous organizations. Knowledge of finance, law, human resources, and related topics improve the systems necessary for the advancement of health care administration and delivery. Nurses are managers, administrators, and executive directors in hospitals, nursing homes, colleges and universities, and health maintenance organizations. Administrators employ, direct, evaluate, promote, and terminate employees. An administrator must have the ability to analyze budgets and make certain that financial plans are consistent with organizational mission and goals. Work hours are often long, but the rewards are gratifying in shaping the future of the organization, the delivery of care, and the profession.

EDUCATIONAL REQUIREMENTS
Bachelor of Science in Nursing is now the entry-level degree. The majority of high-level nursing executives hold a Master of Science in Nursing or an MBA. In addition, many nurse executives are certified in administration through the American Nurses Association Credentialing Center.

CORE COMPETENCIES/SKILLS NEEDED
- Human resource knowledge
- Excellent interpersonal skills
- Ability to communicate clearly and persuasively
- Leadership skills
- Self-confidence
- Budgeting and finance skills
- Writing skills
- Strong work ethic
- Managerial competencies

RELATED WEB SITES AND PROFESSIONAL ORGANIZATIONS
- American Organization of Nurse Executives (www.aone.org)
- American Nurses Association (www.ana.org)
- American College of Healthcare Executives (www.ache.org)

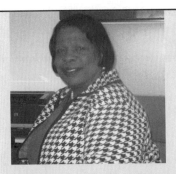

Profile:
LORNA GREEN
Nurse Manager
Gero-Psychiatric Unit

1. What is your educational background in nursing (and other areas) and what formal credentials do you hold?

I am a clinical nurse manager at a major medical center where I have been employed for the past 23 years. My experience includes 9 years as a general duty psychiatric nurse, working with geriatric patients, adult and adolescent patients with various psychiatric diagnoses and symptoms/behaviors, 2 years as senior clinical nurse, and 12 years as a clinical nurse manager. My credentials include an Associate degree in nursing, a Bachelor of Science (Nursing), Cum Laude, and a Master of Science (Nursing).

2. How did you first become interested in the career that you are currently in?

For as long as I can remember, I wanted to be a nurse. During my early childhood, I saw my mother, aunts and neighborhood women minister to friends and relatives who became ill. They provided whatever care was needed for as long as it was needed, without payment or other expectations. All care was rendered at home. Only one doctor was available to provide care for all the people on our island and the nearest hospital was only accessible by boat or by small plane in the later years. Without the diagnosis, care, and support of the neighbors, friends, and relatives, many people would have suffered and died. Therefore, I do not think that I ever "became interested" in nursing, I believe that I was born into it. How fortunate for me that my family, culture, and circumstances of birth allowed me to recognize and develop my passion at a young age. It would not be an exaggeration to state that nursing is not only my profession, it is truly my vocation and one of the most important reasons I am on this earth.

Continued

Profile: LORNA GREEN Continued

3. What are the most rewarding aspects of your career?

Every day in nursing is rewarding in some way for me. Specifically, though, one of the most rewarding days in my life is the day I assumed responsibility of the Geriatric Psychiatry unit. The unit presented a myriad of challenges. Among the most difficult was its reputation for not being consumer oriented and the lack of cohesiveness among staff. Interpersonal relationships were fraught with conflict at times. I am proud to say that through hard work and compromise, we have turned the unit around. We now frequently receive complimentary letters from patients and their families. Doctors, nurses, and other staff members have voiced their appreciation for the improved environment. I take great pride and personal fulfillment in my contributions and continually work hard to seek further enhancements to achieve total consumer and staff satisfaction.

4. What advice would you give to others contemplating a career such as yours?

The most important advice I would impart to a nurse considering a career in administration/management would be to spend the time at the bedside involved in direct patient care as a staff nurse to broaden your knowledge base and gain perspective. Do not jump into the leadership role prematurely. The more you experience and develop, the greater amount of resource will be available to you when you take on additional responsibilities in a leadership role and this will boost your confidence level and others confidence in you when you are making critical decisions.

5 ■ ADULT DAY CARE DIRECTOR

BASIC DESCRIPTION

An adult day care director coordinates, manages, and evaluates care and services to residents of an adult day care program. Residents of adult day care programs are adults who need some assistance in performing activities of daily living such as grooming and other personal care needs. As director of the program, the nurse also monitors the institution's compliance to regulatory standards and is responsible for the oversight of the institution's budget, hiring, and other personnel-related functions.

EDUCATIONAL REQUIREMENTS

Registered nurse preparation and Bachelor of Science in Nursing is required; masters' preparation is highly preferred and at least 3–5 years experience in geriatric nursing is also preferred.

CORE COMPETENCIES/SKILLS NEEDED

- Excellent leadership and management skills
- Knowledge of federal and state regulatory standards that pertain to Adult Day Care management
- Excellent interpersonal and communication skills
- Knowledge of budgeting and fiscal management

RELATED WEB SITE AND PROFESSIONAL ORGANIZATION

- National Adult Day Services Association (http://www.nadsa.org/)

6 ■ ADULT NURSE PRACTITIONER

BASIC DESCRIPTION

Adult nurse practitioners are advanced practice nurses who specialize in providing primary care to adults in a variety of settings, such as hospitals, outpatient clinics, ambulatory care settings, physicians' offices, community-based clinics, and health care agencies. The adult nurse practitioner functions as a primary care provider and focuses on maintaining health and wellness in acute and chronic illnesses. Some of the characteristics of the work are:

- Teaching patients to manage chronic conditions
- Assessing the patient's health history and status
- Ordering diagnostic tests
- Performing therapeutic procedures
- Prescribing medications

EDUCATIONAL REQUIREMENTS

Master of Science in Nursing is required with advanced practice certification as an Adult Nurse Practitioner. Certification as Adult Health Clinical Nurse Specialist, another advanced practice role, is available from the American Nurses Credentialing Center. Graduate programs are generally 2 years in length.

CORE COMPETENCIES/SKILLS NEEDED

- Health assessment skills
- Interpersonal skills
- Ability to work in interdisciplinary teams
- Knowledge of acute and chronic diseases
- Health promotion knowledge and skills
- Knowledge of primary care provider role
- Must possess extensive experience and expertise in assessing and managing patients in primary care settings

RELATED WEB SITES AND PROFESSIONAL ORGANIZATIONS

- American Association of Nurse Practitioners (www.aanp.org)
- Nurse Practitioner Support Services (www.nurse.net)
- Nurse Practitioner Associates for Continuing Education (www.npace.org)
- American Nurses Association Credentialing Center (www.ana.org)
- Nurse Practitioner Programs Directory (www.allnursingschools.com)

7 ■ ADULT PSYCHIATRIC AND MENTAL HEALTH NURSE PRACTITIONER

BASIC DESCRIPTION
Dealing with adult patients, the adult psychiatric and mental health nurse practitioners assess, diagnose, and manage mental health issues that include bipolar disorders, schizophrenia, depression, and anxiety. They may have additional training in psychotherapy or any other behavioral treatment modalities.

EDUCATIONAL REQUIREMENTS
Registered nurse (RN) preparation and Nurse Practitioner certification required. Certification from the American Nurses Credentialing Center also is available as a Clinical Nurse Specialist, another advanced practice nursing specialty role, in psychiatric and mental health; experience as a Mental Health RN is preferred.

CORE COMPETENCIES/SKILLS NEEDED
- Advanced knowledge in mental health
- Sensitivity to patients and their families
- Excellent verbal and written communication skills
- Knowledge in psychopharmacology and behavioral science therapy

RELATED WEB SITES AND PROFESSIONAL ORGANIZATIONS
- American Nurses Credentialing Center (www.nursingcredentialing.org)
- American Psychiatric Nurses Association (www.apna.org)
- International Society of Psychiatric-Mental Health Nurses (http://www.ispn-psych.org/)

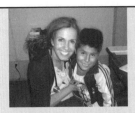

Profile:
MARIANNE TARRAZA
Adult Psychiatric
Mental Health Nurse Practitioner

1. What is your educational background in nursing (and other areas) and what formal credentials do you hold?

My original nursing education was at a hospital-based diploma pro-gram in the Boston area. After receiving my diploma and becoming a registered nurse, I spent several years obtaining my Baccalaureate degree in Nursing (BSN). At that time there were no programs that were designed for an RN to BSN and, subsequently, I had to take many of my original nursing courses for a second time. I ultimately obtained a BSN and quickly moved on to a master's degree in Nursing with a specialization in psychiatric nursing. I am currently certified as an adult psychiatric nurse practitioner.

2. How did you first become interested in the career that you are currently in?

I began my nursing career in medical surgical nursing and psychia-try. I worked primarily as a staff nurse on a large surgical unit and per diem on the psychiatric unit. I then moved on to various surgical disciplines including vascular surgery, intensive care, and noninvasive vascular technology. Since there was a research component to these positions, when I later moved to Maine I worked as the research coordinator in the department of OB/GYN. This position was not nec-essarily what I had chosen but I had young children and this work allowed me the flexibility to care for my children. While participating in clinical research, the nurse in me connected to the lived experi-ences of the patients so much so that when I decided to return for graduate work I returned to my psychiatric roots and concentrated on mental health. I was primarily interested in medical illnesses that were comorbid with psychiatric disorders. I planned on a practice

Continued

Profile: MARIANNE TARRAZA Continued

that was focused primarily on psychotherapy; however, during my training I became increasingly fascinated with psychopharmacology, which now is a significant component in my clinical work.

3. What are the most rewarding aspects of your career?

There are so many rewarding aspects of my career path—it is difficult to say which have been the most rewarding. Even the difficulties within my journey have been rewarding to me since they have led to other aspects that have turned out to be exceptional.

Mental health crosses all disciplines. Whether it is purely a psychiatric disorder, medical comorbidity, or a social/behavioral perspective there is a mental health component. This is the most rewarding aspect of my career. I have the opportunity to examine relationships, coping, behavior, and health from the sphere of the self.

This has also led me to participate in volunteer medical missionary work. I spend time annually working in impoverished areas in South America. The opportunity and, more importantly, the privilege to spend time in these areas have impacted me in a life-changing way. Specifically, how I approach patient care, administrative duties, nursing opportunities, and my own sense of myself have been touched and realigned in a irreplaceable way.

4. What advice would you give to someone contemplating the same career path in nursing?

"Nursing has been good to me" is my favorite personal quote. Nursing has provided me with the opportunity throughout my life to attend to my personal needs while fulfilling my professional promise. I began as a naïve teenager who wanted to "help people" and continue with that mission in mind whenever I take on a new opportunity. It is to that end that I know that I have made an impact on the lives of others even if only for a moment.

There are many avenues in which to consider how to enter nursing, all with strengths and weaknesses. To enter nursing with the

Continued

Profile: MARIANNE TARRAZA Continued

knowledge that there is nothing impossible in this profession, the difference one can make in the lives of others is an endowed privilege. I would suggest having a personal vision that is composed of possibilities now, in the near future, and in the distant future so that nothing that one does at any point is no less than breathtaking!

8 ■ ALLERGY/IMMUNOLOGY NURSE

BASIC DESCRIPTION

An allergy/immunology nurse focuses on the care of patients with chronic allergic conditions. These conditions include asthma, allergic rhinitis, urticaria, and atopic dermatitis. Duties include providing direct patient care and health education and, in most cases, administrative responsibilities such as those of an Allergy Office manager.

EDUCATIONAL REQUIREMENTS

Registered nurse (RN) preparation and Basic Life Support certification are required. An allergy RN can obtain certification in Asthma Education by the National Asthma Educator Certification Board.

CORE COMPETENCIES/SKILLS NEEDED

- Strong assessment and interpersonal skills
- Ability to work with other members of the health care team
- Excellent organizational skills
- Advance knowledge in allergy treatment and management, such as allergy desensitization therapy

RELATED WEB SITES AND PROFESSIONAL ORGANIZATIONS

- American Academy of Allergy, Asthma and Immunology (http://www.aaaai.org/)
- Association of Asthma Educators (http://www.asthmaeducators.org/)
- National Asthma Educator Certification Board (http://www.naecb.org/)

9 ■ AMBULATORY CARE NURSE

BASIC DESCRIPTION

An ambulatory care nurse works as part of a multidisciplinary health care team to provide primary care to a specific population. Depending on the role the nurse plays within the ambulatory center, the work activities will differ. A triage nurse may primarily work in a walk-in area or on the telephone assessing the patients and making determinations on the priority with which they must be seen or referred. Working with a multidisciplinary team entails gathering a medical history and information about the chief complaint and checking vital signs. Once the practitioner has seen the patient, the nurse will perform follow-up treatment such as drawing labs and teaching the patient regarding the condition and discharge instructions.

EDUCATIONAL REQUIREMENTS

Registered nurse preparation is required; certification is available from the American Nurses Credentialing Center.

CORE COMPETENCIES/SKILLS NEEDED

- Knowledge of illnesses and symptoms including diagnosis and management
- Experience with triage
- Strong assessment and organizational skills
- Communication skills
- Ability to collaborate and function as a member of a multidisciplinary team
- Ability to function in a fast-paced environment
- Interest in working with a diverse population

RELATED WEB SITES AND PROFESSIONAL ORGANIZATIONS

- American Academy of Ambulatory Care Nursing (www.aaacn.org/)
- American Nurses Credentialing Center (www.nursecredenting.org)

10 ■ ANTICOAGULATION NURSE

BASIC DESCRIPTION
An anticoagulation nurse is responsible for monitoring patients in ambulatory care settings on anticoagulant therapy such as Coumadin based on clinical standards and protocols. Other responsibilities include anticoagulant medication administration, point-of-care testing, health education to patients and families regarding instructions for medication and care related to anticoagulation therapy.

EDUCATIONAL REQUIREMENTS
Registered nurse license and several years of experience in acute or ambulatory care are required; Basic Life Support certification and completion of Anticoagulation Management Certification Course are highly desirable. Certification is provided by the National Certification Board for Anticoagulation Providers.

CORE COMPETENCIES/SKILLS NEEDED
- Excellent communication skills
- Strong computer skills
- Knowledge of the complex interactions among food, supplements, electrolytes, and drugs with anticoagulant therapy
- Knowledge of physiology of hemostasis and its related pathophysiology

RELATED WEB SITES AND PROFESSIONAL ORGANIZATIONS
- National Certification Board for Anticoagulation Providers (http://www.ncbap.org/)

11 ■ AROMATHERAPIST NURSE

BASIC DESCRIPTION

An aromatherapist nurse is a specially trained nurse who uses the soothing and healing properties of scents from essential oils to relieve pain and other discomforts, decrease stress, elevate moods, relax, and treat conditions. Their services are employed in many health care settings such as health spas, holistic health centers, and hospitals.

EDUCATIONAL REQUIREMENTS

Registered Nurse; certification is preferred; Basic Life Support certification is required.

CORE COMPETENCIES/SKILLS NEEDED

- Knowledge of essential oils and its effects
- Knowledge of Centers for Disease Control infection control principles and standards
- Excellent communication and interpersonal skills

RELATED WEB SITES AND PROFESSIONAL ORGANIZATIONS

- National Association of Holistic Aromatherapy (www.naha.org)
- University of Maryland Center for Integrative Medicine (www.compmed.edu)
- National Center for Complementary and Alternative Medicine (http://nccam.nih.gov/)
- American Holistic Nurses Association (www.ahna.org)

12 ■ ATTORNEY

BASIC DESCRIPTION

Nurse attorneys engage in a range of legal activities including the following:

- Provide legal consult/prosecute/defend cases; may represent individuals, patients, health professionals, or institutions
- Provide depositions and court testimony
- Engage in legal research
- Define standards of care
- Serve as quality-of-care experts for hospitals and other health care institutions
- Review cases
- Define applicable standards of care
- Organize records
- Research the literature
- Provide behind-the-scenes or up-front consultations
- Interview clients and witnesses
- Prepare exhibits
- Prepare questions for depositions and court

EDUCATIONAL REQUIREMENTS

Registered nurse preparation and Juris Doctor degree are required.

CORE COMPETENCIES/SKILLS NEEDED

- Logical thinking skills
- Knowledge of judicial system and health care legislation

RELATED WEB SITES AND PROFESSIONAL ORGANIZATIONS

- The American Association of Nurse Attorneys (www.taana.org)
- Registered Nurse Experts, Inc. (www.rnexperts.com)

13 ■ AUTHOR/WRITER

BASIC DESCRIPTION
An author/writer is a registered nurse who works in any area of writing. This written material may be used in research, biomedical research, education, training, sales and marketing, and other medical mediums and communication forms. Writers need the ability at times to work with voluminous technical information. Authors or editors may write for medical and general interest publications, freelance, professional organizations, and medical trade journals.

EDUCATIONAL REQUIREMENTS
Registered nurse preparation is required; Bachelor of Science in Nursing, or higher, is often also required.

CORE COMPETENCIES/SKILLS NEEDED
- Good command of the English language
- Ability to work alone
- Ability to meet deadlines
- Excellent writing skills
- Health care–related knowledge

RELATED WEB SITES AND PROFESSIONAL ORGANIZATIONS
- Registered Nurse Experts, Inc. (www.rnexperts.com)
- Tips to get published (www.medi-smart.com/authors.htm)
- American Medical Writers Association (www.amwa.org)

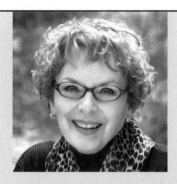

**Profile:
ELEANOR SULLIVAN**
Nurse Author

1. What is your educational background in nursing (and other areas) and what formal credentials do you hold?

I am a nurse author with experience both in nursing and in writing. Following several clinical and teaching positions, I became an associate dean and then a dean of nursing, as well as president of the nursing honor society, Sigma Theta Tau International. My credentials include a PhD, a MSN in psychiatric nursing, a BSN, an ADN, and, more recently, coursework in creative writing.

2. How did you first become interested in the career that you are currently in?

I wrote my first nursing book, *Effective Leadership and Management in Nursing*, because few nursing management books included content from organizational and management literature. That book is now in its eighth edition. Several other nursing books followed, including *Becoming Influential: A Guide for Nurses*, recently released in the second edition.

Like most nurses, I cringed at the inaccurate portrayal of nurses in books, movies, and television. As an avid reader of mysteries, I thought it might be fun to create a story using a nurse sleuth and depict nursing realistically. With my writing background, I thought I could transfer my skills to another genre. I couldn't have been more wrong!

After taking writing courses, attending workshops, and with the help of a talented (and ruthless) editor, my first mystery, *Twice Dead*, featuring nurse sleuth Monika Everhardt was published. Two more books in the series followed, *Deadly Diversion* and *Assumed Dead*,

Continued

Profile: ELEANOR SULLIVAN Continued

and they've been reissued by Harlequin for their mystery line. (See www.EleanorSullivan.com.) All three books will soon be available as e-books.

The success of the nursing mysteries inspired me to try historical fiction based on my family's ancestry. Set in a strict, religious society in 1830s rural Ohio, the stories feature a young midwife in a role anticipating nursing's future. Two books, *Cover Her Body* and *Graven Images*, will be released soon.

3. What are the most rewarding aspects of your career?

Readers' opinions matter most. When people who are not nurses tell me they learned about nursing through my fiction, I feel satisfied that I met my goal. Similarly, nurse readers say that what they learned in *Becoming Influential* they had never been taught in nursing school. Also, I know that my writing will survive me. It is my legacy for the future.

4. What advice would you give to someone contemplating the same career path in nursing?

Read everything you can, especially in the genre that interests you. Attend writers' events, join writers organizations, take writing classes, and write, write, write. Get feedback on your work from other writers who are more experienced than you.

Contrary to popular opinion, writing is hard work. Start small. Write a letter to the editor, comment online about a current news story or offer to review a book for a community publication. Try coauthoring a clinical article with other nurses in your field. There is only one way to success as a writer: persistence. Persistence in learning your craft, persistence in accepting criticism, and persistence in submitting your work to potential markets are all necessary attributes of the published author.

You'll know you're a writer when you receive your first rejection. It won't be your last. Authors who are published didn't let that stop them. Don't let it stop you.

14 ■ BARIATRIC NURSE

BASIC DESCRIPTION
A bariatric nurse provides holistic care to those patients who have a diagnosis of morbid obesity. It also includes care of patients undergoing bariatric surgeries.

EDUCATIONAL REQUIREMENTS
Registered nurse preparation and Basic Life Support certification are required; certification as bariatric nurse is offered by the American Society for Metabolic and Bariatric Surgery.

CORE COMPETENCIES/SKILLS NEEDED
- Excellent assessment and critical thinking skills
- Sensitivity to the needs of patients who are morbidly obese, and their families
- Knowledge of evidence-based practice related to bariatric medicine

RELATED WEB SITES AND PROFESSIONAL ORGANIZATIONS
- National Association of Bariatric Nurses (http://www.bariatric-nurses.org/aboutus.html)
- American Society for Metabolic and Bariatric Surgery (http://www.asbs.org/Newsite07/healthcareprof/alliedhealth/cbn_handbook_2010.pdf)

15 ■ BARIATRIC NURSE PRACTITIONER

BASIC DESCRIPTION

A bariatric nurse practitioner provides either inpatient or outpatient care to patients who are morbidly obese. Aside from providing direct care, a bariatric nurse practitioner provides patient teaching, evaluates patient progress after bariatric surgery and alters plan if needed, and prepares patients for discharge in collaboration with the bariatric surgery team.

EDUCATIONAL REQUIREMENTS

Registered nurse preparation and Nurse Practitioner certification, Basic Life Support certification, and Master of Science in Nursing are required. Advanced training and certification as a bariatric nurse is available by the American Society for Metabolic and Bariatric Surgery and by the American Board of Bariatric Medicine.

CORE COMPETENCIES/SKILLS NEEDED

- Previous experience in bariatric surgery, general surgery, or internal medicine
- Excellent assessment and critical thinking skills
- Sensitivity to the needs of patients who are morbidly obese, and their families
- Knowledge of evidence-based practice related to bariatric medicine

RELATED WEB SITES AND PROFESSIONAL ORGANIZATIONS

- American Board of Bariatric Medicine (http://abbmcertification.org/nurse_practitioners_and_physician_assistants.php)
- National Association of Bariatric Nurses (http://www.bariatric-nurses.org/aboutus.html)
- American Society for Metabolic and Bariatric Surgery (http://www.asbs.org/Newsite07/healthcareprof/alliedhealth/cbn_handbook_2010.pdf)

16 ■ BIOFEEDBACK NURSE

BASIC DESCRIPTION
Biofeedback nurses assist patients to promote and improve health and manage symptoms by using signals from the body. Biofeedback, as a primary treatment modality or as adjunct therapy, is used to manage chronic pain, stress, anxiety, urinary incontinence, asthma, and headache.

EDUCATIONAL REQUIREMENTS
Registered nurse preparation is required; certification is offered by the Biofeedback Certification Institute of America.

CORE COMPETENCIES/SKILLS NEEDED
- Knowledge of operation of equipment used in biofeedback therapy
- Knowledge of the physiologic manifestations of stress, pain, and other chronic conditions
- Excellent interpersonal and communication skills
- Good computer skills and knowledge of electronic health record documentation

RELATED WEB SITES AND PROFESSIONAL ORGANIZATIONS
- Biofeedback Certification Institute of America (www.bcia.org)
- Association for Applied Psychophysiology and Biofeedback (http://www.aapb.org/)

17 ■ BREAST CARE NURSE

BASIC DESCRIPTION

Breast care nurses specialize in caring for patients diagnosed with breast cancer. They provide holistic nursing care that involves assessing breast cancer risks, providing treatment based on a physician's directives, and educating patients with regard to symptom management, psychosocial and spiritual support, and end-of-life care.

EDUCATIONAL REQUIREMENTS

Registered nurse preparation is required; certification is offered by the Oncology Nursing Certification Corporation.

CORE COMPETENCIES/SKILLS NEEDED

- Excellent communication skills
- Ability to provide sensitive care to patients and their families
- Knowledge of resources and agencies for breast cancer patients and survivors
- Knowledge of palliative and end-of-life care
- Knowledge of evidence-based information on breast cancer prevention, care, and management

RELATED WEB SITES AND PROFESSIONAL ORGANIZATIONS

- Oncology Nursing Certification Corporation (http://www.oncc.org/TakeTest/Certifications/CBCN)
- National Breast Cancer Foundation (http://www.nationalbreast-cancer.org/)
- The Breast Cancer Site (http://www.thebreastcancersite.com/clickToGive/home.faces?siteId=2)

18 ■ BURN NURSE

BASIC DESCRIPTION

Nurses who work with burn patients perform comprehensive, highly specialized critical care to adult, geriatric, and pediatric patients who have sustained burn injuries involving up to 100% of total body surface area. The working environment on a burn unit is very intense. The nurse must continually be involved in assessment, planning, and evaluation of care. As part of a highly functioning interdisciplinary team, the nurse must recognize physiological and behavioral changes and know their significance to patient survival. Burn nurses administer pain and other medications, operate special equipment specific to the burn unit, and must maintain fluid and electrolyte balance in their patients.

EDUCATIONAL REQUIREMENTS

Registered nurse preparation is required.

CORE COMPETENCIES/SKILLS NEEDED

Most burn units require 1 year of general medical–surgical or critical care experience, as well as the following:

- Knowledge of the pathophysiology of burns
- Complete understanding of fluid and electrolyte balance
- Technical competency involving complex equipment
- Ability to work with patients on ventilators
- Knowledge of pain management
- Skill in the use of aseptic technique
- Interpersonal competency dealing with patients and families in life-threatening situations
- Ability to work with interdisciplinary teams

RELATED WEB SITES AND PROFESSIONAL ORGANIZATIONS

- American Burn Association (www.ameriburn.org)
- Nurse Friendly (www.nursefriendly.com/burn/)

19 ■ BURN NURSE PRACTITIONER

BASIC DESCRIPTION

A burn treatment nurse practitioner assesses, manages, and evaluates the care of patient in a burn unit. Other responsibilities include health teaching, discharge planning, and coordination of care of patients in a burn unit. Administrative responsibilities include participation in research activities, providing training and lectures at partner institutions or community groups, and participating in quality improvement projects or activities.

EDUCATIONAL REQUIREMENTS

Registered nurse preparation and Nurse Practitioner certification are required; at least 2 to 3 years acute care experience preferably in intensive care unit is highly desired in most positions; Advanced Burn Life Support course is available from the American Burn Association.

CORE COMPETENCIES/SKILLS NEEDED

- Excellent assessment and critical analysis skills
- Excellent interpersonal and communication skills
- Sensitivity to the needs of patients and their families
- Advance knowledge and training in burn and pain management
- Ability to work in a team
- Leadership and organizational skills
- Ability to identify and intervene when critical deviations in patient conditions are noted

RELATED WEB SITES AND PROFESSIONAL ORGANIZATIONS

- American Burn Association (http://www.ameriburn.org)
- Burn Prevention Foundation (http://www.burnprevention.org/)
- Canadian Association of Burn Nurses (http://www.cabn.ca/E-main.php)

20 ■ CAMP NURSE

BASIC DESCRIPTION
A camp nurse provides full health care to children attending camp. In some situations, camps are specific to children with special needs, for example, children with asthma, or children with diabetes. The working environment for a camp nurse is usually one of low stress. Much of the time is spent working with groups of children in an outdoor setting. The work is normally short term during the summer months. However, if a crisis arises, the nurse must have the critical care and rapid response background to deal with life-threatening situations.

EDUCATIONAL REQUIREMENTS
Registered nurse preparation is required.

CORE COMPETENCIES/SKILLS NEEDED
Camp nurses require knowledge of first aid, cardiopulmonary resuscitation, bee stings, snakebites, cuts, and other acute traumatic episodes. Other requirements include

- Understanding separation anxiety
- Interpersonal skills
- First aid knowledge
- Physical and emotional assessment skills
- Medication management
- Ability to respond to unexpected situations

RELATED WEB SITES AND PROFESSIONAL ORGANIZATIONS
- Association of Camp Nurses (www.campnurse.org)
- Camp Nurse Jobs (www.campnursejobs.com)

21 ■ CARDIAC CATHETERIZATION NURSE

BASIC DESCRIPTION

A cardiac catheterization nurse has a specialized role and is a highly skilled cardiovascular nurse whose primary responsibility includes providing nursing care for patients undergoing cardiac catheterization. The spectrum of responsibilities ranges from preadmission to discharge that could include conducting a health screen, preparing patients before the surgery, assisting the surgeon during the surgical procedure, monitoring patients after the surgery, and discharging patients.

EDUCATIONAL REQUIREMENTS

Registered nurse preparation and at least 1 year critical care or emergency room experience is preferred; Advanced Cardiac Life Support and Basic Life Support certifications are required; Critical Care Registered Nurse and/or Registered Cardiovascular Invasive Specialist certification is highly desirable.

CORE COMPETENCIES/SKILLS NEEDED

- Excellent communication skills
- Knowledge of cardiovascular physiology and pathophysiology and cardiac dysrhythmias and their interventions
- Ability to wear lead protection while at work

RELATED WEB SITES AND PROFESSIONAL ORGANIZATIONS

- Cardiovascular Credentialing International (www.cci-online.org)
- American Association of Critical Care Nurses (www.aacn.org)
- Johnson and Johnson Discover Nursing campaign (http://www. discovernursing.com/jnj-specialtyID_255-dsc-specialty_detail.aspx)

22 ■ CARDIOTHORACIC INTENSIVE CARE NURSE

BASIC DESCRIPTION
A cardiothoracic intensive care nurse works in a highly specialized cardiothoracic intensive care unit (ICU) catering to the needs of patients requiring constant monitoring and whose clinical conditions are considered critical. The cardiothoracic intensive care nurse is adept at noting subtle hemodynamic changes that could lead to serious complications and providing immediate interventions as required. The ICU nurse is comfortable in operating and managing complex medical equipment such as ventilators and telemetry monitors and works closely with physicians and unlicensed assistive personnel. The cardiothoracic intensive care nurse usually takes care of no more than two acutely ill patients in a shift.

EDUCATIONAL REQUIREMENTS
Registered nurse preparation, Basic Life Support certification, and Advanced Cardiac Life Support certification are required; certification as critical care registered nurse is available from the American Association of Critical Care Nurses.

CORE COMPETENCIES/SKILLS NEEDED
- Ability to work in a dynamic and intense environment that requires quick thinking and excellent analytical and assessment skills
- Strong background knowledge on hemodynamics, arrhythmia management, pathophysiology, and pharmacology
- Excellent interpersonal and communication skills
- Excellent technical skills such as intravenous management and ventilator care
- Strong computer skills needed for electronic health record documentation
- Strong leadership and delegation skills

RELATED WEB SITE AND PROFESSIONAL ORGANIZATION
- American Association of Critical Care Nurses (http://www.aacn.org/)

23 ■ CARDIOTHORACIC INTENSIVE CARE NURSE PRACTITIONER

BASIC DESCRIPTION

A cardiothoracic intensive care nurse practitioner provides primary care to adults who have acute and complex cardiovascular conditions that require constant monitoring. The cardiothoracic intensive care nurse practitioner works in a highly specialized acute care unit that caters to the needs of patients who have undergone coronary artery bypass graft surgery, heart valve replacement, pacemaker and internal defibrillator placement, heart and lung transplants, and other major cardiothoracic surgeries.

EDUCATIONAL REQUIREMENTS

Registered nurse preparation and Nurse Practitioner certification, master's degree in nursing or higher, and Basic Life Support and Advanced Cardiac Life Support certifications are required; certification as acute care nurse practitioner is offered by the American Association of Critical Care Nurses and American Nurses Credentialing Center.

CORE COMPETENCIES/SKILLS NEEDED

- Excellent assessment and decision-making skills
- Advanced knowledge in hemodynamic pathophysiology, assessment, diagnosis, management, and pharmacology
- Strong leadership and organizational skills
- A high level of stress tolerance and the ability to work in fast-paced and highly dynamic environments
- Ability to work autonomously
- Could be involved in unit- or hospital-based clinical research

RELATED WEB SITES AND PROFESSIONAL ORGANIZATIONS

- American Association of Critical Care Nurses (http://www.aacn.org/)
- American Nurses Credentialing Center (http://www.nursecredentialing.org/)

24 ■ CARDIOTHORACIC NURSE ANESTHETIST

BASIC DESCRIPTION
A cardiothoracic nurse anesthetist works in collaboration with anesthesiologists to provide anesthesia care to patients undergoing heart transplants, ventricular remodeling, and cardiothoracic operations.

EDUCATIONAL REQUIREMENTS
Registered nurse preparation and certification as certified registered nurse anesthetist are required; Basic Life Support and Advanced Cardiac Life Support certifications are also required; experience in acute or emergency care is required as a prerequisite to most positions; certification is offered by the National Board on Certification and Recertification of Nurse Anesthetists.

CORE COMPETENCIES/SKILLS NEEDED
- Excellent interpersonal and communication skills
- Excellent assessment skills and advance knowledge in cardiovascular, pulmonary, and hemodynamic physiology, management, and pharmacology
- Ability to work in a high-stress environment that requires quick decision making
- Strong computer and documentation skills and knowledge of electronic health record

RELATED WEB SITES AND PROFESSIONAL ORGANIZATIONS
- American Association of Nurse Anesthetists (http://www.aana.com/)
- International Federation of Nurse Anesthetists (http://ifna-int.org/ifna/news.php)
- National Board on Certification and Recertification of Nurse Anesthetists (http://www.nbcrna.com/)

25 ■ CARDIOVASCULAR NURSE

BASIC DESCRIPTION
The cardiovascular nurse works with patients who have compromised cardiovascular systems. Cardiac nurses perform postoperative care on a surgical unit, stress test evaluations, cardiac monitoring, vascular monitoring, and health assessments. The setting can be varied depending on the focus of the patient population. Cardiovascular nurses can work in acute care settings with surgical patients, in outpatient clinics doing case management, and in home care.

EDUCATIONAL REQUIREMENTS
Registered nurse preparation is required; certification as cardiovascular nurse is available from the American Nurses Credentialing Center and as a critical care nurse from the American Association of Critical Care Nurses.

CORE COMPETENCIES/SKILLS NEEDED
- Basic Life Support and Advanced Cardiac Life Support certifications
- Proficiency in reading cardiac monitors
- Critical care experience
- Knowledge of cardiac rhythms and cardiac disease
- Good interpersonal skills
- Ability to work with interdisciplinary teams
- Ability to manage acute episodes in chronically ill patients

RELATED WEB SITES AND PROFESSIONAL ORGANIZATIONS
- American Association of Cardiovascular and Pulmonary Rehabilitation (www.aacvpr.org)
- National Association of Vascular Access Networks (www.navannet.org)
- American Nurses Credentialing Center (www.nursecredentialing.org)
- Society for Vascular Nursing (www.svnnet.org)
- American Association of Critical Care Nurses (www.aacn.org)

26 ■ CASE MANAGER

BASIC DESCRIPTION
Case management is the process of organizing and coordinating resources and services in response to individual health care needs along the illness and care continuum in multiple settings. There are many models for case management based on client, context, or setting. The nurse case manager assesses and monitors clients and the health care delivery services that they require. Case management is directed toward a targeted or selected client/family population such as transplant, head-injured, or frail elderly clients. The goals are to center services around the patient, to foster patient self-managed care, and to maximize efficient and cost-effective use of health resources. The focus is cost saving and continuity of care. Case managers have the opportunity to work in hospitals, community outreach, clinics, occupational health, insurance companies, and health maintenance organizations.

EDUCATIONAL REQUIREMENTS
Registered nurse preparation and Bachelor of Science in Nursing are required; master's degree is preferred; certification in case management is available from the American Nurses Credentialing Center.

CORE COMPETENCIES/SKILLS NEEDED
- Strong knowledge base in both the financial and clinical aspects of care
- Understanding of community resources
- Strong communication skills
- Effective skills in managing, teaching, and negotiating
- Ability to work with interdisciplinary groups
- Ability to focus on patients and families

RELATED WEB SITES AND PROFESSIONAL ORGANIZATIONS
- The American Association of Managed Care Nurses (www.aamcn.org)
- Commission for Case Manager Certification (www.ccmcertification.org)
- Case Management Society of America (www.cmsa.org)

27 ■ CHEMOTHERAPY NURSE

BASIC DESCRIPTION
Chemotherapy nursing is a specialty within oncology nursing. Chemotherapy nurses administer and monitor the patient receiving chemotherapeutic agents as ordered by physicians. Working closely with oncologists and pharmacists, their job responsibilities could also include obtaining patient histories, collecting specimens, evaluating effectiveness of treatment, and educating patients on treatment and follow-up care.

EDUCATIONAL REQUIREMENTS
A registered nurse license is required, and Bachelor of Science in Nursing is preferred; Basic Life Support certification is required, and Advanced Cardiac Life Support certification is preferred; certification as Oncology Certified Nurse could be obtained by passing a certification examination offered by the Oncology Nursing Society's Oncology Nursing Certification Corporation. For recertification, 1,000 hours of clinical practice in oncology and continuing professional development activities are required.

CORE COMPETENCIES/SKILLS NEEDED
- Excellent intravenous skills including starting, maintaining, and troubleshooting common intravenous access problems
- Excellent communication skills and organizational skills
- Knowledge of cancer, its pathophysiology, and common treatments and side effects

RELATED WEB SITES AND PROFESSIONAL ORGANIZATIONS
- Oncology Nursing Society (www.ons.org)
- Johnson and Johnson Discover Nursing (http://www. discovernursing.com/jnj-specialtyID_117-dsc-specialty_detail.aspx)
- Association of Pediatric Hematology Oncology Nurses (www.aphon.org)

28 ■ CHILD ADOLESCENT PSYCHIATRIC MENTAL HEALTH CLINICAL NURSE SPECIALIST

BASIC DESCRIPTION

A child adolescent psychiatric mental health clinical nurse specialist (CNS) is an advanced practice nurse who works with children and adolescents with psychiatric problems, focusing on the individual client/patient with any presenting health problem. The advanced practice role is aimed at early intervention and treatment of children with mental illness, and includes use of a wide range of psychotherapeutic skills (e.g., individual, family, and group therapy). The child adolescent psychiatric mental health CNS practices in both inpatient and outpatient hospital settings and a variety of other settings such as clinics, schools, community agencies, day treatment facilities, and public health departments. Additional advanced practice activities include consultation to other professional and nonprofessional groups and education of other professionals, administrators, and researchers.

EDUCATIONAL REQUIREMENTS

Registered nurse preparation and licensure; advanced practice licensure; and master's, postmaster's, or doctoral preparation in a CNS program in child/adolescent psychiatric mental health nursing are required. Advanced practice certification requires a minimum of 500 supervised clinical hours in the specialty. Certification from the American Nurses Credentialing Center is available.

CORE COMPETENCIES/SKILLS NEEDED

- Advanced assessment skills
- Advanced knowledge of pharmacology and pathophysiology
- Ability to meet the child at his or her developmental level
- Clinical skill in at least two psychotherapeutic treatment modalities

- Ability to facilitate coordination and collaboration among agencies delivering care to children
- Ability to provide services to children and their families
- Flexibility and sensitivity

RELATED WEB SITES AND PROFESSIONAL ORGANIZATIONS

- Association of Child and Adolescent Psychiatric Nurses Division, International Society of Psychiatric-Mental Health Nurses (http://www.ispn-psych.org/html/acapn.html)
- American Psychiatric Nurses Association (www.apna.org)
- American Nurses Credentialing Center (http://www.nursecredentialing.org/Eligibility/ChildAdolescentPsychCNS.aspx)

29 ■ CHILD PSYCHIATRIC NURSE

BASIC DESCRIPTION

A child psychiatric nurse is one who works with children and adolescents with psychiatric problems and who focuses on the entire continuum between health and illness. The nurse's role is aimed at promotion and prevention, early intervention, and treatment of children with mental illness. The child psychiatric nurse practices in a variety of settings such as clinics, schools, community agencies, psychiatric hospitals, day treatment facilities, and public health departments. Generalist activities of a child psychiatric nurse include teaching parents with emotionally disturbed or mentally retarded children or adolescents; participation as a member of a health care delivery team, and participation in research activities related to the field of child and adolescent psychiatric nursing.

EDUCATIONAL REQUIREMENTS

Registered nurse preparation and licensure, with certification in psychiatric/mental health nursing, are required.

CORE COMPETENCIES/SKILLS NEEDED

- Ability to meet the child at his or her developmental level
- Knowledgeable about psychiatric mental health treatment and services
- Ability to facilitate coordination and collaboration among agencies delivering care to children
- Ability to provide services to children and their families
- Flexibility and sensitivity

RELATED WEB SITES AND PROFESSIONAL ORGANIZATIONS

- American Psychiatric Nurses Association (www.apna.org)
- Association of Child and Adolescent Psychiatric Nurses Association (www.ispn-psych.org/html/acapn.html)
- American Nurses Credentialing Center (http://www.nursingworld.org/ancc/index.htm)

30 ■ CHILDBIRTH EDUCATOR

BASIC DESCRIPTION

The childbirth educator provides informational and educational classes for expectant parents. Classes include information on relaxation techniques, comfort measures, breathing techniques, and birth options. Childbirth educators play an important role in the emotional, physical, and informational support for expectant parents. Most hospitals and birthing centers offer this type of educational program for their clients. Usually, a nurse with excellent teaching and interpersonal skills is selected to teach class on-site to expectant parents.

EDUCATIONAL REQUIREMENTS

Registered nurse preparation is required; certification may be obtained through the Childbirth and Postpartum Professional Association.

CORE COMPETENCIES/SKILLS NEEDED

- Must have knowledge about the childbearing years, pregnancy, and labor and delivery
- Teaching ability
- Clinical competence in obstetrical nursing
- Interpersonal skills
- Collaboration with physicians

RELATED WEB SITES AND PROFESSIONAL ORGANIZATIONS

- Childbirth Organization (www.childbirth.org/)
- Childbirth and Postpartum Professional Association (www.cappa.net)
- Lamaze International (www.lamaze.com/)

31 ■ CIRCULATING NURSE

BASIC DESCRIPTION

The circulating nurse, an integral part of the perioperative team, serves as an advocate for patients who are under anesthesia and/or sedation. Responsibilities include ensuring that surgical asepsis is adhered to during the surgical procedure, keeping track and conducting an inventory of supplies and equipment used during and after the surgical procedure, or calling for a time-out. The Joint Commission has specified a "time-out" immediately before surgery to prevent surgical errors.

EDUCATIONAL REQUIREMENTS

Registered nurse licensure is required; Advanced Cardiac Life Support and Basic Life Support certifications are mostly required for this position; Certified Nurse Operating Room certification is highly desirable.

CORE COMPETENCIES/SKILLS NEEDED
- Excellent communication skills
- Ability to work with members of the perioperative team
- Excellent observation skills
- Knowledge of asepsis, infection control, and effects of anesthesia

RELATED WEB SITE AND PROFESSIONAL ORGANIZATION
- Association of Perioperative Registered Nurses (www.aorn.org)

32 ■ CLINICAL NURSE SPECIALIST

BASIC DESCRIPTION
The clinical nurse specialist coordinates activities regarding patient care on a specific unit within the hospital. This is an advanced practice role and requires a Master of Science in Nursing. The setting is usually inpatient hospital, and intense. Clinical nurse specialists (CNS) assist the multidisciplinary team from admission to discharge; answer and refer questions the family might have; are involved in health teaching and support/counseling; assist in developing protocols for managing care of the client; serve as a resource person to staff nurses and other health team members; collect data and investigate trends for the program, for example, heart surgery; facilitate discharge preparation for a smooth transmission back home; and coordinate follow-up visits for the patient.

EDUCATIONAL REQUIREMENTS
Registered nurse preparation and Master of Science in Nursing are required. Most settings require 5 years of acute care experience. Certification in various CNS roles is available from the American Association of Critical Care Nursing and American Nurses Credentialing Center.

CORE COMPETENCIES/SKILLS NEEDED
- Self-confidence and strong leadership skills
- Excellent communication
- Understanding of organizational structure
- Technical competency involving use of complex equipment
- Teaching skills
- Clinical competency
- Ability to work with interdisciplinary teams
- Skills in staff evaluation

RELATED WEB SITES AND NURSING ORGANIZATIONS

- National Association of Clinical Nurse Specialists (www.nacns.org)
- American Board of Nursing Specialties (www.nursingcertifica-tion.org)
- American Nurses Credentialing Center (www.nursingworld.org/ancc/index.htm)
- American Association of Critical Care Nurses (http://www.aacn.org/wd/certifications/content/ccnslanding.pcms?menu=certification)

33 ■ CLINICAL RESEARCH NURSE

BASIC DESCRIPTION

A clinical research nurse works in clinical research centers and acts as a patient advocate in ensuring that ethical and efficient care is provided in compliance with federal and local research regulations. Their nursing knowledge provides them with the unique opportunity to meet the complex needs of patients participating in a research study.

EDUCATIONAL REQUIREMENTS

Registered nurse preparation, Bachelor of Science in Nursing, and Basic Life Support certification are required; recent acute care experience is required in most positions.

CORE COMPETENCIES/SKILLS NEEDED

- Knowledge of research process and evidence-based nursing
- Knowledge of Institutional Regulatory Board policies
- Excellent interpersonal and communication skills
- Good computer skills and knowledge of electronic health record

RELATED WEB SITES AND PROFESSIONAL ORGANIZATIONS

- Association of Clinical Research Professionals (http://www.acrp-net.org/)
- Society of Clinical Research Associates (www.socra.org)

34 ■ COMMUNITY HEALTH NURSE

BASIC DESCRIPTION
A community health nurse is someone who delivers nursing care for individuals and families where they live, work, or go to school. The community health nurse may or may not have education and training in public health nursing. The practice settings for the community health nurse are varied and include home care, school-based care, and occupational health care.

EDUCATIONAL REQUIREMENTS
A registered nurse license is required and at least 1 year of acute care experience is required for most jobs; certification is provided by the American Nurses Credentialing Center.

CORE COMPETENCIES/SKILLS NEEDED
- Excellent assessment and communication skills
- Good clinical and analytical skills
- Ability to travel to many locations
- Strong computer skills especially in using portable devices for documentation
- Excellent organization and management skills

RELATED WEB SITES AND PROFESSIONAL ORGANIZATIONS
- Association of Community Health Nursing Educators (www.achne.org)
- American Nurses Credentialing Center (www.nursecredentialing.org)
- American Public Health Association (www.apha.org)

35 ■ COMPLIANCE SPECIALIST NURSE

BASIC DESCRIPTION

A compliance specialist nurse's primary responsibility is to review medical record claims for a health care organization to assess accuracy of services and quality of care provided, and to assess whether these services have met practice and ethical standard requirements. He or she provides the review team with her clinical expertise in investigating a case.

EDUCATIONAL REQUIREMENTS

Registered nurse preparation, Bachelor of Science in Nursing, and at least 3 years of clinical experience, preferably in home care, are desired in most job positions.

CORE COMPETENCIES/SKILLS NEEDED

- Experience in utilization review, risk management, and quality management
- Strong background in clinical compliance, medical record review, and documentation
- Knowledge of CPT and ICD-9 codes
- Understanding of Medicare and Medicaid regulations
- Must be ethical, objective, detail oriented, and able to work in a high-stress environment
- Strong computer skills and knowledge and data management skills
- Excellent communication, organizational, and interpersonal skills

RELATED WEB SITE AND PROFESSIONAL ORGANIZATION

- Ethics and Compliance Officer Association (http://www.theecoa.org/iMIS15/ECOAPublic/)

36 ■ CONSULTANT

BASIC DESCRIPTION

A consultant is one who gives advice or provides specialized services on an hourly or contractual basis; nurse consultants can provide advice and/or services in a wide range of areas, such as research development, clinical areas of expertise (diabetes, cardiovascular disease), curriculum development, staffing of health care institutions, and so forth. A consultant might work or practice in virtually any and all aspects of the health care industry, including private practice. Health care in general and nursing in particular provide a wide range of opportunities for consultants. Services can be provided as part of a group effort or by an individual with a specific area of expertise.

EDUCATIONAL REQUIREMENTS

Registered nurse preparation is required; often additional education is required in the consultant's area of expertise. For example, research consultants would have PhD degrees and clinical consultants would have graduate degrees in their clinical area of specialization.

CORE COMPETENCIES/SKILLS NEEDED

- Independent functioning and team skills, with a clear focus on results that are contracted for by the client
- Entrepreneurial skills
- Communication skills
- Organizational skills
- Writing ability
- Leadership skills
- Project management skills

RELATED WEB SITE AND PROFESSIONAL ORGANIZATION

- National Nurses in Business Association (www.nnba.net)

37 ■ CONTINENCE NURSE

BASIC DESCRIPTION
The continence nurse—a specialty role—is responsible for assessing, planning, intervening, and evaluating care of patients who have urinary and/or fecal incontinence.

EDUCATIONAL REQUIREMENTS
Registered nurse license and a minimum of a Bachelor of Science in Nursing are required; certification as Certified Continence Nurse is available from the Wound, Ostomy, and Continence Certification Board.

CORE COMPETENCIES/SKILLS NEEDED
- Strong assessment and verbal and written communication skills
- Knowledge of anatomy, physiology, and pathophysiology of the genitourinary and gastrointestinal systems
- Strong computer skills and some knowledge in data collection and interpretation
- May be involved in establishing care protocols and processes of care that relate to the care of patients with continence issues

RELATED WEB SITE AND PROFESSIONAL ORGANIZATION
- Wound, Ostomy, and Continence Nursing Certification Board (www.wocncb.org)

38 ■ CORONARY CARE NURSE

BASIC DESCRIPTION

A coronary care nurse specializes in the care of patients who have acute and chronic coronary conditions requiring close assessment and monitoring. They also provide essential care in the patient's cardiac rehabilitation program. They need to be familiar with electrocardiogram rhythms, emergency cardiac care, and cardiovascular medications.

EDUCATIONAL REQUIREMENTS

Registered nurse preparation is required; Bachelor of Science is required in most positions; Basic Life Support and Advanced Cardiac Life Support certifications are also required; certification in Cardiac Vascular Nursing is offered by the American Nurses Credentialing Center and the American Association of Critical Care Nurses.

CORE COMPETENCIES/SKILLS NEEDED

- Ability to work in a fast-paced environment that requires quick decision making
- Excellent communication, analytical, and assessment skills
- Strong background knowledge of cardiovascular pathophysiology and pharmacology
- Strong computer skills needed for electronic health record documentation
- Strong leadership and delegation skills

RELATED WEB SITES AND PROFESSIONAL ORGANIZATIONS

- American Association of Cardiovascular and Pulmonary Rehabilitation (http://www.aacvpr.org/)
- Society for Vascular Nursing (http://www.svnnet.org/)
- American Nurses Credentialing Center (http://www.nursecredentialing.org/NurseSpecialties/CardiacVascular.aspx)
- American Association of Critical Care Nurses (www.aacn.org)

39 ■ CORRECTIONAL FACILITY NURSE

BASIC DESCRIPTION

The nurse who works in a correctional facility provides health care for all inmates. This includes case management, responding to episodes of acute illness, emergency call management, psychiatric evaluations, and assessment of new inmates. The patients are those with health problems related to chronic illness, AIDS, substance abuse, renal failure/dialysis, respiratory diseases, and terminal cancer.

EDUCATIONAL REQUIREMENTS

Registered nurse preparation is required. Positions are entry level, and orientation and assignment to a preceptor is required in most correctional facilities.

CORE COMPETENCIES/SKILLS NEEDED

The nurse who works in a correctional facility needs strong basic nursing skills, including:

- The ability to function independently
- The ability to respond to emergency situations
- Knowledge of mental health issues
- Health promotion and disease prevention skills
- Strong assessment skills

RELATED WEB SITE AND PROFESSIONAL ORGANIZATION

- Official Home of Corrections (www.corrections.com)

40 ■ CRITICAL CARE NURSE

BASIC DESCRIPTION

A critical care nurse cares for patients who are critically ill. The nurse has a great deal of one-on-one contact with the patient and is often the main source of contact for the family members. A critical care nurse is responsible for constant monitoring of the patient's condition, as well as recognition of any subtle changes. These nurses use a large amount of technology within their practice and function as integral members of the multidisciplinary health care team. Critical care nurses must possess the ability to collaborate with other members of the health care team such as physicians, case managers, therapists, and, especially, other nurses. They are responsible for all care given to the patient, from medication administration to tracheotomy and other ventilator care, as well as constant monitoring of the patient for any alterations in their status. Responsibilities include monitoring, assessment, vital sign monitoring, ventilatory management, medication administration, intravenous insertion and infusion, central line care, Swan-Ganz catheters, and maintenance of a running record of the patient's status. He or she must be prepared at all times to perform cardiopulmonary resuscitation and other lifesaving techniques.

EDUCATIONAL REQUIREMENTS

Registered nurse preparation and Advanced Cardiac Life Support certification are required. Bachelor of Science in Nursing and Critical Care Nurse certification are preferred, and may be required depending on the institution. Most institutions require at least 1 to 2 years of medical/surgical experience, although some hospitals are offering extended preceptorships to selected new graduates. Previous critical care experience is desired. In addition to prior experience, many institutions require nurses to pass a critical care course, usually offered in the hospital, and to complete 4 to 6 weeks of orientation to the unit. Certification in critical care or cardiac medicine is available from the American Association of Critical Care Nursing Certification Corporation.

CORE COMPETENCIES/SKILLS NEEDED

- Excellent assessment skills, ability to detect very subtle changes in a patient's condition
- Strong organizational skills, ability to prioritize
- Communication skills and patient and family education skills
- Strong knowledge of anatomy and physiology, medications and their actions, interactions, side effects, and calculations
- Maturity and ability to handle end-of-life issues such as when to cease life-prolonging interventions or organ donation decisions
- An affinity for technology

RELATED WEB SITE AND PROFESSIONAL ORGANIZATION

- American Association of Critical-Care Nurses (www.aacn.org)

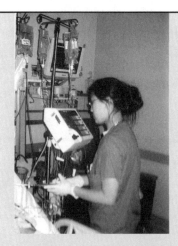

Profile:
MAY LING LUC
Critical Care Nurse

1. What is your educational background in nursing (and other areas) and what formal credentials do you hold? (no need to indicate the schools where you received the degrees)

I have a bachelor's degree in nursing and am a certified critical care nurse (CCRN).

2. How did you first become interested in the career that you are currently in?

The career found me. I originally majored in physical therapy in college; however, I lost interest in it and became exploratory for a semester until my advisor told me to try out nursing. She called the assistant dean of the school of nursing. I had a meeting with her, she looked at my credentials and said that I should transfer to the school of nursing. I did, and that summer I found out that I was going to be a nursing student. It was one of the best things that ever happened to me. I love doing what I do.

3. What are the most rewarding aspects of your career?

When patients are truly appreciative of what I do for them.

4. What advice would you give to someone contemplating the same career path in nursing?

Observe first, if you have a close friend who is a nurse, get his/her aspect of it. Also go for either your bachelor's or master's degree in nursing.

41 ■ CRITICAL CARE TRANSPORT NURSE

BASIC DESCRIPTION

The critical care transport nurse (CCTN) provides essential services in ensuring the safe on-ground transfer of acutely ill patients from one health care facility to another. The CCTN assesses, monitors, intervenes, and stabilizes critically ill patients during transport.

EDUCATIONAL REQUIREMENTS

A registered nurse license and at least 2 years of critical care or emergency room experience are required; current Basic Life Support, Advanced Cardiac Life Support, and Pediatric Advanced Life Support certifications are required; certification as Certified Transport Registered Nurse is available from the Emergency Nurses' Association Board of Certification for Emergency Nursing.

CORE COMPETENCIES/SKILLS NEEDED
- Ability to work in a high-stress environment
- Ability to lift or move objects over 80 pounds
- Excellent communication and assessment skills
- Strong computer skills and ability to use electronic health record/ documentation effectively
- Strong clinical, critical thinking, and decision-making skills

RELATED WEB SITES AND PROFESSIONAL ORGANIZATIONS
- Air and Surface Transport Nurses Association (www.astna.org)
- Emergency Nurses Association (www.ena.org)

42 ■ CRUISE SHIP/RESORT NURSE

BASIC DESCRIPTION

Cruise ship/resort nurses work on ships or at resorts to provide emergency and general care to passengers/vacationers, should it be required. These nurses also serve as part of the occupational health team for crew members who live on the ship for 6 to 8 months at a time, or for the staff at resorts. Responsibilities include providing patient care in the health center and dealing with on-site emergencies. This work offers flexibility. Assignments are 3- to 6-month contract positions, living and working with the same people, and meeting people from around the world.

RESPONSIBILITIES INCLUDE

- Providing patient care both on a day-to-day basis and in emergency situations
- Maintaining rapport with guests, physicians, and other crew members
- Communicating to arrange for workers or guests to receive medical attention
- Providing discharge instructions for each patient
- Preparing and maintaining medical records and billing for all patients
- Complying with resort and maritime rules, regulations, and procedures

EDUCATIONAL REQUIREMENTS

Registered nurse preparation with a minimum of 2 years of recent hospital experience is required. Experience with cardiac care, trauma, and internal medicine is desirable.

CORE COMPETENCIES/SKILLS NEEDED

- Excellent interpersonal skills; must enjoy traveling and must be flexible
- Excellent communication skills
- Strong health assessment skills
- A valid passport
- Ability to advise patients with colds, headaches, or other minor illnesses

RELATED WEB SITES AND PROFESSIONAL ORGANIZATIONS

- Cruise Line Employment (www.cruiselinejob.com/medical.htm)
- Nursing Spectrum Career Fitness Online; *Cruising to a New Opportunity*, by Pat Clutter, RN, MEd, CEN (http://nsweb. nursingspectrum.com/cfforms/cruising.cfm)

43 ■ DEAN OF NURSING

BASIC DESCRIPTION

The dean of nursing is an administrative position in a school or college of nursing. Aside from providing academic and educational leadership to the faculty, students, and alumni, he/she supervises faculty-related procedures that relate to instructional, research, and service programs; oversees the budgetary needs; and conducts evaluations of associate and assistant deans and chairs of the department/college of school.

EDUCATIONAL REQUIREMENTS

A master's degree or higher is required.

CORE COMPETENCIES/SKILLS NEEDED

- Strong administrative, interpersonal, and communication skills
- Strong background in organizational leadership and management, fiscal and budgetary affairs, and nursing research and education
- Knowledge of nursing curriculum and university/college policies
- Strong background in human resources–related matters

RELATED WEB SITES AND PROFESSIONAL ORGANIZATIONS

- American Associations of Colleges of Nursing (http://www.aacn.nche.edu/ContactUs/index.htm)
- National League for Nursing (http://www.nln.org/)

44 ■ DERMATOLOGY NURSE PRACTITIONER

BASIC DESCRIPTION

The dermatology nurse practitioner—an advanced practice role—is responsible for assessing, diagnosing, and treating common dermatological disorders such as psoriasis, dermatitis, or eczema and dermatological infections such as those caused by viruses, fungi, or bacteria.

EDUCATIONAL REQUIREMENTS

A master's degree and Nurse Practitioner certification are required; for certification as a Dermatology Certified Nurse Practitioner, a minimum of 3,000 hours of practice in dermatology and a Nurse Practitioner certification are required.

CORE COMPETENCIES/SKILLS NEEDED

- Excellent assessment skills
- Advanced knowledge of the physiology and pathophysiology in dermatology and their treatment
- Ability to work with collaborating dermatologist

RELATED WEB SITES AND PROFESSIONAL ORGANIZATIONS

- Dermatology Nursing (www.dermatologynursing.net)
- Nurse Practitioner Society of Dermatology Nurses' Association (www.dnanurse.org)

45 ■ DERMATOLOGY NURSE

BASIC DESCRIPTION
This multifaceted job encompasses the full spectrum of patient care of those who have dermatological conditions. Dermatology nurses work in clinics, hospitals, and other health care settings. The job responsibilities include skin cancer screening, assistance in treatment, administrative work, and patient teaching.

EDUCATIONAL REQUIREMENTS
A registered nurse license is highly preferred; an initial 3-year certification is available from the Dermatology Nursing Certification Board, a member of the American Board of Nursing Specialties.

CORE COMPETENCIES/SKILLS NEEDED
- Excellent organizational and communication skills
- Knowledge of the physiology and pathophysiology in dermatology, and their treatment
- Continuing education credits is required for recertification

RELATED WEB SITES AND PROFESSIONAL ORGANIZATIONS
- Dermatology Nursing (www.dermatologynursing.net)
- Dermatology Nurses' Association (www.dnanurse.org)

46 ■ DEVELOPMENTAL DISABILITIES NURSE PRACTITIONER

BASIC DESCRIPTION

Developmental disabilities nurse practitioners are clinical experts in providing primary care to those who have cognitive and physical disabilities such as mental retardation, autism, and Asperger's syndrome. Developmental disabilities nurse practitioners are also strong advocates in fostering improved knowledge about the care of patients who have developmental disabilities. They are employed in various settings such as hospitals, schools, and primary care centers.

EDUCATIONAL REQUIREMENTS

Registered nurse license, Nurse Practitioner certification, and Basic Life Support certification are required; certification as a developmental disabilities nurse is required in most positions.

CORE COMPETENCIES/SKILLS NEEDED

- Excellent communication and assessment skills
- Strong advocate for and commitment to the issues that relate to the care of patients who have developmental disabilities
- Strong computer and documentation skills
- Sensitivity to the unique needs of patients with developmental/learning disabilities and their families

RELATED WEB SITE AND PROFESSIONAL ORGANIZATION

- Developmental Disabilities Nurses Association (www.ddna.org)

47 ■ DIABETES EDUCATOR

BASIC DESCRIPTION
The diabetes educator works with diabetic patients to teach them about diabetes and how to live a healthy life with this very common health problem. Most diabetic educators work in clinics or physician offices and manage the care of clients with this disease. The diabetic nurse educator establishes long-term commitments and knows patients very well. Responsibilities include instruction on foot and skin care, and appropriate diet; monitoring of blood glucose; and administration of insulin. The diabetic educator must have knowledge of hypoglycemia and hyperglycemia, and must keep up with the newest techniques and interventions available.

EDUCATIONAL REQUIREMENTS
The care of diabetic patients is very complex and requires a minimum of a Bachelor of Science in Nursing and special certification as a diabetic educator. Increasingly, Master of Science in Nursing preparation is required. Certification is available from the National Certification Board for Diabetes Educators.

CORE COMPETENCIES/SKILLS NEEDED
■ Extensive expertise and knowledge about the care of diabetic patients, patient education skills, and interpersonal skills

RELATED WEB SITES AND NURSING ORGANIZATIONS
■ American Association of Diabetes Educators (www.aadenet.org)
■ National Certification Board for Diabetes Educators (www.ncbde.org)

48 ■ DIALYSIS NURSE

BASIC DESCRIPTION
A dialysis nurse—a specialized role in nephrology nursing—specifically provides care to patients undergoing dialysis or peritoneal dialysis. Dialysis is a life-saving and/or -sustaining procedure performed in patients who have kidney failure.

EDUCATIONAL REQUIREMENTS
Registered nurse preparation is required; Bachelor of Science in Nursing is highly preferred and Basic Life Support certification is required; certification as either nephrology or dialysis nurse is available from the Board of Nephrology Examiners Nursing and Technology or from the Nephrology Nursing Certification Commission.

CORE COMPETENCIES/SKILLS NEEDED
- Knowledge and familiarity of equipment used for hemodialysis and peritoneal dialysis
- Strong interpersonal, communication, assessment, and analytical skills
- Sensitivity to patient needs and their families

RELATED WEB SITES AND PROFESSIONAL ORGANIZATIONS
- American Nephrology Association (www.annanurse.org)
- Nephrology Nursing Certification Commission (www.nncc-exam.org)
- Board of Nephrology Examiners Nursing and Technology (www.bonent.org)

49 ■ DISASTER/BIOTERRORISM NURSE

BASIC DESCRIPTION
The disaster/bioterrorism nurse works in disaster areas that are the result of a bioterrorist attack or in situations caused by natural disaster, war, or poverty. Red Cross nurses are often part of the network that provides assistance during times of disaster or conflict. The nature of the work will vary depending on the course of the disaster or conflict.

EDUCATIONAL REQUIREMENTS
Registered nurse preparation is required. Red Cross nurses must have special training and 20 hours of volunteer or paid service before being assigned to a disaster situation.

CORE COMPETENCIES/SKILLS NEEDED
- Emergency room or critical care experience
- Experience with local disaster action teams
- Management skills
- Ability to meet the needs of people in crisis and high-stress situations
- Knowledge of disaster preparedness and basic first aid

RELATED WEB SITES AND PROFESSIONAL ORGANIZATIONS
- American Red Cross (www.redcross.org)
- American Nurses Association: Bioterrorism and Disaster Response (www.nursingworld.org/news/disaster/)

50 ■ DOMESTIC VIOLENCE NURSE EXAMINER

BASIC DESCRIPTION

These specialists are trained not only to care for patients who are survivors of domestic violence but also to spot signs of abuse and to accurately document evidence that could be used in legal proceedings. They work in various health care settings such as emergency departments, ambulatory settings, shelters, and in advocacy groups that serve domestic violence victims. They could also be trained mental health counselors or sexual assault nurse examiners (SANE).

EDUCATIONAL REQUIREMENTS

Registered nurse preparation is required; Bachelor of Science in Nursing is preferred; certification as SANE is preferred in most job positions; SANE certification is offered by the Forensic Nursing Certification Board.

CORE COMPETENCIES/SKILLS NEEDED

- Advance knowledge in forensics and preparation as mental health counselor
- Excellent verbal and written communication skills
- Ability to provide sensitive and culturally appropriate care to victims of abuse
- Knowledge of resources and agencies that provide care and assistance to domestic violence victims

RELATED WEB SITES AND PROFESSIONAL ORGANIZATIONS

- Nursing Network on Violence Against Women, International (http://www.nnvawi.org/)
- International Association of Forensic Nursing (www.iafn.org)

51 ■ EAR, NOSE, AND THROAT NURSE

BASIC DESCRIPTION
Nurses in this area of practice deal with patients who have ear, nose, and throat (ENT) conditions. They work in various health care settings and cater to all patient populations. They could work in outpatient ENT clinics that cater to minor ENT problems or in special units that cater to complex ENT cases such as those with maxillofacial trauma or those undergoing head and neck surgeries and chemotherapy.

EDUCATIONAL REQUIREMENTS
Registered nurse preparation is required; specialty certification is offered by the National Certifying Board of Otorhinolaryngology and Head–Neck Nurses.

CORE COMPETENCIES/SKILLS NEEDED
- Knowledge of ENT pathophysiology and its management
- Excellent interpersonal skills and sensitivity to the needs of patients who may have body image issues
- Strong computer skills and knowledge of electronic health record
- Ability to work in a team

RELATED WEB SITE AND PROFESSIONAL ORGANIZATION
- Society of Otorhinolaryngology and Head–Neck Nurses (http://www.sohnnurse.com/ent.html)

52 ■ EAR, NOSE, AND THROAT NURSE PRACTITIONER

BASIC DESCRIPTION

Ear, nose, and throat nurse practitioners diagnose, treat, and evaluate patients who have ear, nose, and throat (ENT) disorders. Other primary responsibilities include ordering diagnostic tests, providing health promotion education, assisting the surgeon in ENT surgeries, and evaluating patient progress and discharging patients as appropriate.

EDUCATIONAL REQUIREMENTS

Registered nurse preparation and Nurse Practitioner certification are required.

CORE COMPETENCIES/SKILLS NEEDED

- Advanced knowledge related to ENT pathophysiology and disease diagnosis, and medical–surgical and pharmacological management of patients who have ENT conditions
- Excellent interpersonal and communication skills
- Ability to work in a team
- Sensitivity to the needs of patients and their families and knowledge of resources and referral networks available

RELATED WEB SITE AND PROFESSIONAL ORGANIZATION

- Society of Otorhinolaryngology and Head–Neck Nurses (http://www.sohnnurse.com/ent.html)

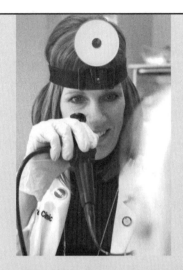

Profile:
ERIN ROSS
ENT Nurse Practitioner

1. What is your educational background in nursing (and other areas) and what formal credentials do you hold?

I received a Bachelor of Science in Nursing, a master's degree in nursing, and am currently enrolled in a professional doctoral program (DNP). I am certified as an otorhinolaryngology and head–neck nurse, and am a certified nurse practitioner (NP). I have over 21 years of nursing experience.

2. How did you first become interested in the career that you are currently in?

I first became interested in ear, nose, and throat (ENT) nursing while working in the operating room (OR) and intensive care unit (ICU) at a major medical center. I began working with a prominent head and neck surgeon as a nurse clinician in his medical practice. He began to mentor and train me as he would have prepared a medical resident. My experience as an OR nurse helped me to assist in the OR during cases. I made rounds with the doctor, co-wrote orders, and assisted with the in-house patients. On the outpatient side, I was available in the office to triage calls, manage patients going through surgery, and performed small office procedures (removal of nasal packing, stitches, gave chemical peels, etc). When I began my nurse practitioner training, he mentored me to another level. I began

Continued

Profile: ERIN ROSS Continued

to do flexible nasal scoping, laryngoscopy, earwax removal, sinus/ nasal debridements, and simple biopsies. He showed me the side to managing a patient practice. I was responsible for ordering supplies and working with office assistants. He encouraged me to join a professional nursing organization. I began to attend nursing meetings, moved on to giving lectures, became a coordinator of an ENT nursing review course, and was elected to the board of directors. I am happy to say I am now the vice president of my professional nursing organization, the Society of Otorhinolaryngology and Head–Neck Nurses.

3. What are the most rewarding aspects of your career?

I enjoy three things: empowering my patients to live a healthy lifestyle and helping them when they are not; teaching others about ENT nursing; and the flexibility that is offered by nursing and my position. I am able to have a balance with my professional life and family.

4. What advice would you give to someone contemplating the same career path in nursing?

I would tell someone to follow their instincts. Nursing is not a "catch all" profession. I would not tell someone to go into it for the money or the stability of a job. Go into nursing to give something back. Nursing can allow you many opportunities. I have worked in the OR, the ICU, a medical surgical floor, as a liver/kidney procurement coordinator, a preceptor, adjunct faculty, and—the best one of all—an ENT NP. I have a great professional career, which has been balanced with family life. Many times I have been asked why I did not become a doctor, I simply reply "because I love being a nurse." I found what I was meant to do. I have never looked back. No regrets.

53 ■ EDITOR, BOOK

BASIC DESCRIPTION
This is a nurse who edits books and/or monographs for publication in print or through electronic media. The work may be in any scientific/professional content area in nursing and health care or related areas. This edited material may be used in research, education, training, sales and marketing, and other mediums and communication forms. The editor can be the originator of the content idea for the book, or can be hired by others to do the editing work. This specialty combines editing and writing skills with nursing and health care knowledge. There are numerous opportunities for freelance work that can be done from home with flexible hours. Sometimes the work can be isolating and the data can be very technical, detail oriented, tedious, and voluminous; however, the work varies depending on the content being edited. Opportunities exist to work for nursing and medical marketing/communications companies, pharmaceutical companies, nursing, medical and general interest publishing houses, nursing and medical education companies, and professional organizations.

EDUCATIONAL REQUIREMENTS
Registered nurse preparation is required; Bachelor of Science in Nursing, or higher, is often required; content expertise is expected.

CORE COMPETENCIES/SKILLS NEEDED
- Excellent writing skills
- Good command of the English language
- Attention to detail
- Strong organizational and analytical skills
- Ability to work alone
- Ability to meet deadlines
- Excellent computer skills
- Health care–related knowledge

RELATED WEB SITES AND PROFESSIONAL ORGANIZATIONS

- International Academy of Nurse Editors (http://www.nursingeditors-inane.org/)
- Nurse Author Editor (http://www.nurseauthoreditor.com/)
- American Medical Writers Association (www.amwa.org)
- American Copyeditors Society (http://www.copydesk.org/)
- Board of Editors in the Life Sciences (http://www.bels.org/)

54 ■ EDITOR, JOURNAL

BASIC DESCRIPTION
This is a nurse who edits journals of other periodical publications, published in print or through electronic media. The work may be in any scientific/professional content area in nursing and health care or related areas. This edited material may be used in research, education, training, sales and marketing, and other mediums and communication forms. The editor of the journal/periodical is usually selected and contracted by the publishing company or professional organization that owns the publication. The editor is most often selected for both content expertise and editing/publication experience. This specialty combines editing and writing skills with nursing and health care knowledge. There are numerous opportunities for freelance work that can be done from home with flexible hours. Sometimes the work can be isolating and the data can be very technical, detail oriented, tedious, and voluminous; however, the work varies depending on the content being edited. Opportunities exist to work for major publishing companies in the health sciences, nursing and medical marketing/communications companies, pharmaceutical companies, general interest publishing houses, nursing and medical education companies, and professional organizations.

EDUCATIONAL REQUIREMENTS
Registered nurse preparation is required; Bachelor of Science in Nursing, or higher, is often required; content expertise is expected.

CORE COMPETENCIES/SKILLS NEEDED
- Excellent writing skills
- Good command of the English language
- Attention to detail
- Strong organizational and analytical skills
- Ability to work alone

- Ability to meet deadlines
- Excellent computer skills
- Health care–related knowledge
- Ability to work with others, for example, editorial board members, association board members

RELATED WEB SITES AND PROFESSIONAL ORGANIZATIONS

- International Academy of Nurse Editors (http://www.nursingeditors-inane.org/)
- Nurse Author Editor (http://www.nurseauthoreditor.com/)
- American Medical Writers Association (www.amwa.org)
- American Copyeditors Society (http://www.copydesk.org/)
- Board of Editors in the Life Sciences (http://www.bels.org/)
- Committee on Publication Ethics (http://publicationethics.org/)
- International Committee of Medical Journal Editors (http://www.icmje.org/)
- Council of Science Editors (http://www.councilscienceeditors.org)
- American Society of Healthcare Publication Editors (http://www.ashpe.org/)

55 ■ EDUCATOR

BASIC DESCRIPTION

College and university faculty who teach and advise students on basic and graduate degree programs in nursing are nurse educators or academic nurses. Faculty may give lectures to several hundred students in large halls, lead small seminars, or supervise students in laboratories. They prepare lectures, exercises, and laboratory experiments; grade exams and papers; and advise and work with students individually. In universities, they also supervise graduate students' teaching and research. Faculty members are expected to keep up with developments in their field by reading current literature and participating in professional conferences. Faculty members consult with government, business, nonprofit, and community organizations. They also do their own research to expand knowledge in their field. They perform experiments; collect and analyze data; and publish their research results in professional journals, books, and electronic media. Most faculty members serve on academic or administrative committees that deal with the policies of their institution, departmental matters, academic issues, curricula, budgets, equipment purchases, and hiring. Some work with student and community organizations. Department chairpersons are faculty members who usually teach some courses but have heavier administrative responsibilities. Clinical faculty members provide clinical supervision of students.

EDUCATIONAL REQUIREMENTS

Requirements vary with level of position; college faculty and deans usually need a doctorate (PhD, EdD, DNSc, DNP); these individuals serve as the top administrative officer of the academic unit for full-time, tenure-track positions in 4-year colleges and universities; instructors and clinical faculty most often have educational preparation at the master's degree level. Certification is available from the National League for Nursing.

CORE COMPETENCIES/SKILLS NEEDED
- Strong interpersonal and communication skills
- Motivational and mentoring skills
- Knowledge of teaching/learning and/or management principles and practices
- Ability to make sound decisions and to organize and coordinate work efficiently
- Time management skills; ability to work independently and manage a large number of diverse projects
- Research and publication skills, especially for faculty at professorial ranks in colleges and universities
- Ability to manage a flexible schedule; faculty usually teach 12 to 16 hours per week, and for faculty and committee meetings. Most faculty establish regular office hours for student consultations, usually 3 to 6 hours per week. Faculty devote time to course preparation, grading, research, graduate student supervision, and other activities.

RELATED WEB SITES AND PROFESSIONAL ORGANIZATIONS
- National League for Nursing (www.nln.org)
- American Association of Colleges of Nursing (www.aacn.nche.edu)

56 ■ ELECTROPHYSIOLOGY NURSE

BASIC DESCRIPTION
An electrophysiology nurse—a specialty in cardiology nursing—assists and educates patients undergoing an electrophysiology study procedure of the heart. An electrophysiology study of the heart involves a nonsurgical procedure to obtain information about the heart's electrical activity. They also work with patients who have pacemakers or defibrillators.

EDUCATIONAL REQUIREMENTS
Registered nurse preparation and Basic Life Support and Advanced Cardiac Life Support certifications are required; certification is available from the American Nurses Credentialing Center as a Cardiac/Vascular Nurse and from the American Association of Critical Care Nurses as a critical care nurse.

CORE COMPETENCIES/SKILLS NEEDED
- Minimum acute care experience preferably in emergency nursing or critical care
- Strong knowledge in cardiology
- Excellent assessment and critical thinking skills

RELATED WEB SITES AND PROFESSIONAL ORGANIZATIONS
- American Nurses Credentialing Center (http://www. nursecredentialing.org/NurseSpecialties/CardiacVascular.aspx).
- Preventive Cardiovascular Nurses Association (http://www.pcna.net/)
- American Association of Critical Care Nurses (www.aacn.org)

57 ■ EMERGENCY ROOM NURSE

BASIC DESCRIPTION

Emergency department (ED) or emergency room (ER) nurses specialize in trauma and critical care, working in environments that are specially equipped to manage emergency care in life-threatening circumstances. ED nurses are often on the front line of health care, as many persons use the ER as their primary source of care.

EDUCATIONAL REQUIREMENTS

Registered nurse preparation with 1 to 3 years of acute care experience. Although not required by all ERs, ED nurses are usually trained in advanced cardiac support and pediatric advanced life support. Certification is available from the Board of Certification for Emergency Nursing.

CORE COMPETENCIES/SKILLS NEEDED

- Organization skills
- Ability to triage patients
- Mental ability to deal with death and dying
- Ability to take medical histories and make accurate assessments quickly
- Ability to manage mass casualty situations
- Technical proficiency with health care equipment
- Ability to function in high-stress situations

RELATED WEB SITES AND PROFESSIONAL ORGANIZATIONS

- Emergency Nurses Association (www.ena.org)
- Willy's Emergency Nursing Web (www.virtualnurse.com/er/er.html)

58 ■ EMERGENCY ROOM NURSE PRACTITIONER

BASIC DESCRIPTION

The emergency room nurse practitioner—an advanced practice role—delivers primary care in the emergency department. They could treat common urgent and nonemergency medical conditions in collaboration with the emergency room attending physician.

EDUCATIONAL REQUIREMENTS

Registered nurse preparation, Nurse Practitioner certification, and Master of Science in Nursing are required; previous experience in emergency room or critical care nursing is often required for the position; certification as acute care nurse practitioner is offered by the American Nurses Credentialing Center and by American Association of Critical Care Nurses.

CORE COMPETENCIES/SKILLS NEEDED
- Excellent analytical and communication skills
- Advanced training and education in the care of critically ill patients
- Ability to work under pressure and make quick important clinical decisions
- Excellent management and organization skills and ability to work with members of the health care team
- Strong computer skills especially in the use of electronic health record/documentation

RELATED WEB SITES AND PROFESSIONAL ORGANIZATIONS
- American Nurses Credentialing Center (www.nursecredentialing.org)
- American Association of Critical Care Nurses (www.aacn.org)
- American College of Nurse Practitioners (www.acnp.org)

59 ■ ENDOCRINOLOGY NURSE

BASIC DESCRIPTION
An endocrinology nurse is someone who specializes in the care of patients who have endocrine disorders such as diabetes mellitus and Cushing's disease. They work across age groups and they are employed in various health care settings such as inpatient hospital units or departments or ambulatory centers. Some endocrinology nurses also specialize, such as a pediatric endocrinology nurse.

EDUCATIONAL REQUIREMENTS
Registered nurse preparation is required. Bachelor of Science in Nursing is highly preferred; Basic Life Support certification is required.

CORE COMPETENCIES/SKILLS NEEDED
- Strong knowledge of the endocrine system and hormonal system
- Excellent interpersonal, communication, assessment, and analytical skills
- Sensitivity to the needs of patients and their families
- Strong computer skills, including the use of electronic health record documentation
- Ability to work in a team
- Strong organizational and leaderships skills especially for those who have administrative duties commonly found in ambulatory endocrine centers

RELATED WEB SITES AND PROFESSIONAL ORGANIZATIONS
- Endocrine Nurses Society (www.endo-nurses.org)
- Society for Endocrinology (www.endocrinology.org)
- Pediatric Endocrinology Nursing Society (www.pens.org)
- American Diabetes Association (www.diabetes.org)

60 ■ ENDOSCOPY NURSE

BASIC DESCRIPTION
The endoscopy nurse is responsible for providing nursing care for those patients, of all age groups, undergoing endoscopic procedures; they are employed in various settings such as ambulatory centers or inpatient endoscopy units.

EDUCATIONAL REQUIREMENTS
Registered nurse license and current Basic Life Support certification are required, and most facilities require at least 2 years of acute care experience. Most positions require certification in gastroenterology available from the American Board for Gastroenterology Nurses.

CORE COMPETENCIES/SKILLS NEEDED
- Ability to physically assist patients during endoscopic procedures that could include lifting, bending, pushing, and pulling
- Adequate manual dexterity
- Knowledge of basic electrocardiogram rhythms and dysrhythmia and effects of sedation
- Ability to effectively communicate with patients and with members of the interprofessional team
- Strong computer and documentation skills

RELATED WEB SITE AND PROFESSIONAL ORGANIZATION
- American Board for Gastroenterology Nurses (www.cgrn.com)

61 ■ ENDOSCOPY NURSE PRACTITIONER

BASIC DESCRIPTION

The endoscopy nurse practitioner provides primary care to those patients undergoing endoscopic procedures. Aside from performing or assisting in endoscopy, they also provide post-procedure follow-up and patient education, and discharge patients once stable.

EDUCATIONAL REQUIREMENTS

Registered nurse preparation, Nurse Practitioner certification, and Basic Life Support/Advanced Cardiac Life Support certification are required; acute clinical experience as a registered nurse is also required; certification as a gastroenterology nurse and training in gastroenterology medicine are required in most job positions.

CORE COMPETENCIES/SKILLS NEEDED

- Excellent assessment and analytical skills
- Ability to sit or stand in the endoscopy suite for an extended period of time and ability to physically assist patients with lifting, bending, pushing, or pulling
- Strong leadership and organizational skills
- Advanced knowledge related to the physiology, pathophysiology, and pharmacological management of the gastrointestinal system
- Ability to effectively communicate with patients and with members of the interprofessional team

RELATED WEB SITE AND PROFESSIONAL ORGANIZATION

- American Board for Gastroenterology Nurses (www.cgrn.com)

62 ■ ENTREPRENEUR

BASIC DESCRIPTION
An entrepreneur is a nurse who starts his/her own business, assuming all risk and responsibility. These entrepreneurs may work in any aspect of the health care/medical industry. Examples of settings include both independent practice or corporations and industry.

EDUCATIONAL REQUIREMENTS
Registered nurse license is required. Bachelor of Science in Nursing and Master of Science in Nursing are desired. Degree in business is helpful.

CORE COMPETENCIES/SKILLS NEEDED
- Must possess desire to have own business and/or practice independently
- Excellent communication skills
- Independent individual who is flexible, autonomous, and has creative freedom
- Self-motivated, ambitious, determined, and self-confident
- Willing to take risks and make important decisions

RELATED WEB SITES AND PROFESSIONAL ORGANIZATIONS
- National Nurses in Business Association (www.nnba.net)
- US Small Business Administration (www.sba.gov)

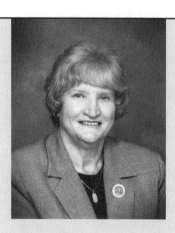

Profile:
JEAN AERTKER
Nurse Entrepreneur

1. What is your educational background in nursing (and other areas) and what formal credentials do you hold?

I began my professional nursing career in 1973 with an Associate Degree in Nursing (ASN) and was one of the few commissioned into the United States Air Force (USAF) Nurse Corps with the ASN degree; I was commissioned in 1974. I completed the Baccalaureate in Nursing (BSN) degree and then pursued a Masters in Nursing with a nurse practitioner focus. I completed a professional doctorate (DNP) in 2008. I am Board Certified Nurse Practitioner.

2. How did you first become interested in the career that you are currently in?

While serving as an officer in the USAF Nurse Corps in 1974, I was introduced to the then evolving role of the nurse practitioner. While the role seemed limited to pediatrics and women's health in the early years, nurse practitioners began to work more in the outpatient primary care clinics and family practice areas. The opportunity to promote health and wellness before illness or chronic disease states erupted seemed the best fit for my future nursing career and interest.

3. What are the most rewarding aspects of your career?

The reward of extensive education and leadership opportunities gave me the confidence to be a successful nurse entrepreneur and build my own practice by 1998. With this independence of ownership, I

Continued

Profile: JEAN AERTKER Continued

have a greater flexibility to be a mentor and consultant to new nurse practitioners and nursing colleagues in the industry. My role enables me to be more visible as an expert nurse in the community and in the workplace. It is a privilege to represent nursing through a business perspective.

4. What advice would you give to someone contemplating the same career path in nursing?

The educational ladder beginning with an associate degree in nursing has value for those who plan to enter the world of work in nursing promptly, but it should not end there. I consider it the first rung on the ladder from which to build and develop the necessary skills and knowledge to care for today's patient in a very complex health care system. Many educational options face the nursing student today and they can be very confusing. The program of choice must meet the needs of the student, their family, and the community which includes the nursing profession. Nursing has long debated the appropriate degree for the entry level into professional nursing, but whatever route the student chooses, they must know there are many personal rewards in achieving the highest level of education in order to serve others and the profession.

63 ■ EPIDEMIOLOGY NURSE

BASIC DESCRIPTION

A nurse epidemiologist investigates trends in groups or aggregates and studies the occurrence of diseases and injuries. The information is gathered from census data, vital statistics, and reportable disease records. Nurse epidemiologists identify people or populations at high risk; monitor the progress of diseases; specify areas of health care need; determine priorities, size, and scope of programs; and evaluate their impact. They generally do not provide direct patient care, but serve as a resource and plan educational programs. They also publish results of studies and statistical analysis of morbidity and mortality. Examples of practice settings are the Centers for Disease Control and Prevention in Atlanta, Georgia; public health departments; and governmental agencies.

EDUCATIONAL REQUIREMENTS

Masters degree in Public Health or Community Health Nursing is required. A PhD is preferred.

CORE COMPETENCIES/SKILLS NEEDED

- Must possess mathematical and analytical ability
- Knowledge of both infectious and noninfectious diseases
- Desire to improve the health and well-being of populations
- Ability to identify populations at risk
- Knowledge of health policy
- Must plan programs and health services

RELATED WEB SITES AND PROFESSIONAL ORGANIZATIONS

- Centers for Disease Control and Prevention (www.cdc.gov)
- Association for Professionals in Infection Control and Epidemiology, Inc. (www.apic.org)

64 ■ ETHICIST

BASIC DESCRIPTION
An ethicist is a nurse who knows about legal/moral/ethical issues and provides services for patients and families. The nurse ethicist may work with an ethics team to develop a detailed investigative plan to answer questions raised by an ethics violation allegation or resolve ethical dilemmas. Opportunities exist to work in hospitals, nursing homes, hospices, and outpatient settings.

EDUCATIONAL REQUIREMENTS
Registered nurse preparation and Master of Science in Nursing or graduate degree in bioethics or a related field are required.

CORE COMPETENCIES/SKILLS NEEDED
- Requires technical training and previous experience with investigations
- Excellent communication skills
- Involves conducting and documenting investigations
- May include interviewing and/or reviewing documents that may pertain to the allegations
- Knowledge of ethical and legal issues surrounding end-of-life care
- Knowledge of compliance-related concepts, policies, and procedures
- Must be able to work well with others to draw conclusions based on allegations
- Expertise in pain management and issues of loss and grief are helpful

RELATED WEB SITES AND PROFESSIONAL ORGANIZATIONS
- Nursing Ethics Network (www.nusingethicsnetwork.org/)
- Nursing World Ethics (www.nusingworld.org/ethics/)
- Hospice Foundation of America (www.hospicefoundation.org/)

65 ■ FAMILY NURSE PRACTITIONER

BASIC DESCRIPTION
Family nurse practitioners (FNPs) are advanced practice nurses who specialize in providing health promotion and care to patients in primary care settings. The FNP provides primary screenings and focuses on health promotion and disease prevention across the life span. FNPs have many of the same duties as acute care practitioners, but typically do not work with patients who are critically ill. FNPs perform physical examinations, order diagnostic tests, establish diagnoses, prescribe medications, and educate patient and family members regarding health and illness conditions and treatment plans. Examples of settings in which an FNP might practice are physicians' offices, health care clinics, private practice, hospitals, long-term care facilities, public health departments, and occupational health settings.

EDUCATIONAL REQUIREMENTS
Master of Science in Nursing with advanced practice certification as an FNP is required. Programs are generally 2 years in length combining clinical and didactic work. Certification is available from the American Nurses Credentialing Center.

CORE COMPETENCIES/SKILLS NEEDED
- Ability to perform physical examinations
- Ability to assess accurately when doing screenings and diagnostic tests; knowledge of normal ranges and abnormal findings
- Strong communication skills
- Teaching ability and interest
- Ability to work with interdisciplinary teams as well as to function independently

- Knowledge of acute and chronic conditions
- Excellent judgment in knowing when to make a referral
- Prescribing of medications

RELATED WEB SITES AND PROFESSIONAL ORGANIZATIONS

- American Academy of Nurse Practitioners (www.aanp.org)
- American College of Nurse Practitioners (www.nurse.org/acnp)
- American Nurses Credentialing Center (www.nursecredentialing. org)

66 ■ FAMILY PSYCHIATRIC/MENTAL HEALTH NURSE PRACTITIONER

BASIC DESCRIPTION
Family psychiatric nurse practitioners work with families to provide a full range of mental health care that includes assessing, diagnosing, and managing mental health issues. They may possess advanced training in psychotherapy, symptom management and psychopharmacology. They treat various conditions that include bipolar disorders, schizophrenia, depression and anxiety.

EDUCATIONAL REQUIREMENTS
RN Preparation and NP certification; Certification from the American Nurses Credentialing Center is available; experience as a Mental Health RN is preferred in most positions.

CORE COMPETENCIES/SKILLS NEEDED
- Advanced knowledge in mental health
- Sensitivity to patients and their families
- Excellent verbal and written communication skills
- Strong computer and documentation skills
- Ability to work as a member of a team

RELATED WEB SITES AND PROFESSIONAL ORGANIZATIONS
- American Nurses Credentialing Center (www.nursing credentialing.org)
- American Nurses Psychiatric Nurses Association (www.apna.org)
- International Society of Psychiatric-Mental Health Nurses (http://www.ispn-psych.org/)

67 ■ FIRST ASSIST NURSE

BASIC DESCRIPTION
The registered nurse first assist (RNFA) works alongside with the surgeon during the perioperative phase. The RNFA has undergone additional training to help surgeons in preoperative skin preparation, controlling surgical site bleeding, suturing, cutting, and cleansing surgical areas and applying dressings.

EDUCATIONAL REQUIREMENTS
A registered nurse license, Certified Nurse Operating Room certification, completion of post-basic nursing study that meets Association of periOperative Registered Nurses (AORN) standards for an RNFA education program, Basic Life Support certification, and successful passing of the Certified Registered Nurse First Assistant certification examination are required for practice. Certification is also available from the Competency and Credentialing Institute.

CORE COMPETENCIES/SKILLS NEEDED
- Excellent communication skills
- Significant experience and knowledge in perioperative nursing
- Ability to work collaboratively with members of the perioperative team

RELATED WEB SITES AND PROFESSIONAL ORGANIZATIONS
- Association of periOperative Registered Nurses (http://www.aorn.org)
- Registered Nurses First Assist Home (http://www.rnfa.org)
- Competency and Credentialing Institute (http://www.cc-institute.org)

68 ■ FLIGHT NURSE/CRITICAL CARE TRANSPORT

BASIC DESCRIPTION
A flight nurse is a highly trained and experienced critical care registered nurse (RN). The flight nurse works with a flight crew most likely consisting of the flight nurse/paramedic, flight respiratory therapist/EMT-1, and a pilot to transport patients to, from, and between hospital facilities. Flight nurses work in intensive care units, emergency rooms, ambulance companies, and emergency transport facilities.

EDUCATIONAL REQUIREMENTS
Bachelor of Science in Nursing required. She/he must hold current certification as a Certified Flight RN, Certified Emergency Nurse, or Certified Critical Care Nurse and be certified as a paramedic. Advanced Cardiac Life Support and Pediatric Advanced Life Support, Neonatal Advanced Life Support, completion of a trauma nurse core curriculum, and completion of a flight nurse advanced trauma course are needed. This usually requires a minimum of 2 to 3 years of critical care nursing experience. Rigorous ongoing continuing education is necessary to support the extensive knowledge and skills that are expected for flight nurses.

CORE COMPETENCIES/SKILLS NEEDED
- Experience in multisystem trauma; neonates; pediatrics; severe burns; acute medical, high-risk obstetrics; and cardiac patients
- Prepared to use endotracheal intubations and chemical paralytic agents; must be prepared for the placement of central venous access via the femoral or subclavian route, surgical airways, pericardiocentesis, needle thoracostomy, and intraosseous access
- Assume responsibility for sharing knowledge about emergency care systems with other members of the health care team, patients, their significant others, and the community

- Involved in research that directly relates to improved patient care in the air medical transport industry, and/or improves the professional standards of practice that promote the flight nurse as a professional
- Responsible for direct patient care during transport, which may include monitoring, medication administration, assessment, intravenous infusion, ventilatory/airway management, charting, and communication with other health care providers
- Provide the rapid assessment, diagnosis, and treatment of critically injured or ill patients of all ages from the scene of an accident or from referring facilities

RELATED WEB SITES AND PROFESSIONAL ORGANIZATIONS

- Air and Surface Transport Nurses Association (www.astna.org)
- Board of Certification for Emergency Nursing (www.ena.org/bcen)

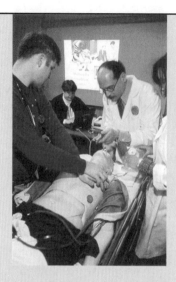

Profile:
CHRISTOPHER MANACCI
Flight Nurse

1. What is your educational background in nursing (and other areas) and what formal credentials do you hold?

I hold a master's degree in nursing and am currently enrolled in a professional doctoral program (DNP). I am an acute care nurse practitioner. I also am the founding director of the world's first university-based graduate program in flight nursing. I maintain a full-time critical care practice as the managing nurse practitioner of critical care transport at a major medical center where I am responsible for operational and clinical practice oversight. My practice in the air medical arena spans nearly three decades. I put into practice the first critical care air rescue and evacuation service, utilizing acute care nurse practitioners. This model places the diagnostician and the prescribing clinician at the side of patient during a turbulent time of transition. I have held faculty appointments as Consulting Professor of Critical Care, Department of Navy, Special Warfare, and a Subject Matter Expert for NASA.

2. How did you first become interested in the career that you are currently in?

I first became interested in flight nursing while I was practicing in the intensive care unit (ICU) at a large community-based hospital. I enjoyed the complexity of the ICU patient population, but desired to

Continued

Profile: CHRISTOPHER MANACCI Continued

practice in an environment that required more acute intervention and stabilization. I transitioned to the emergency department of an urban level-1 trauma center. After several years of practice, I missed the sophistication of the ICU patient population. Flight nursing combines the sophistication of an intensive care unit with the urgency of an emergency department. It seemed like the "best of both worlds" as I was looking to increase my level of practice and capability.

3. What are the most rewarding aspects of your career?

I provide advanced practice nursing care, such as assessment, planning, and independent prescriptive intervention based on real-time diagnostic data. In addition, I provide advanced procedures of airway management, central line placement, tube thoracostomy, and emergent surgical interventions when dictated by the clinical presentation. Preplanning for the unknown is the common denominator in flight nursing advanced practice. There is no way to anticipate what type of mission awaits you, but a mission of some type is certain. I have completed as many as seven helicopter missions in a 12-hour shift. As a program with three online Sikorsky S 76-A++ helicopters, four Citation V Ultra jet aircraft, and two specially configured surface transport vehicles, our program has completed as many as 26 missions in a 24-hour period. I believe that there are many dimensions to each individual existence that transcend the interpretation of their reality, to which humility and grace can alter the course of destiny. Also, I believe that the difference between difficult and impossible is a matter of education, interpretation, and intervention. Enhancement of the human condition is the practice of nursing.

4. What advice would you give to someone contemplating the same career path in nursing?

Every specialty in nursing provides you with unique opportunities, but flight nursing, especially in an advanced practice role provides you with all of them. It is necessary to have a strong clinical background in critical care nursing and a strong understanding of pathophysiology, pharmacology, and clinical management of a variety of disease

Continued

93

Profile: CHRISTOPHER MANACCI Continued

processes. It is essential that you enjoy caring for critically ill patients in unstructured environments and austere conditions. The best candidate is a clinically proficient individual who is formally educated and trained in the notions of autonomous and collaborative practice. I believe it is helpful if you have completed research related to the care of individuals in suboptimal conditions and have the ability to evaluate and implement necessary changes in therapeutic interventions. Gain as much education and knowledge as early in your career as possible; do not jump from unit to unit, rather develop clinical depth in the process of caring for patients. This coupled with clinical expertise and skill proficiencies will provide you with the ability to be a strong candidate for a flight nursing position at a staff level or as an advanced practice nurse. Most importantly this will provide you with the tools to care for your patients in any setting. The most important asset is the desire to make a difference and the passion to alter the destiny of those entrusted to your care.

69 ■ FORENSIC NURSE

BASIC DESCRIPTION
Forensic nurses combine clinical nursing practice in conjunction with knowledge of law enforcement. They provide care to victims and are involved in the investigation of sexual assault, elder and spousal abuse, and unexplained or accidental death. Forensic nursing is high stress because of the nature of the work, and it requires a broad understanding of social, environmental, and psychological influences on behavior. The environments in which forensic nurses work are varied. They work in such settings as correctional institutions, psychiatric facilities, acute care settings, coroner and medical examiners' offices, and for insurance companies.

EDUCATIONAL REQUIREMENTS
Registered nurse preparation and Bachelor of Science in Nursing are required; often, graduate preparation is required. Certification from Sexual Assault Nurse Examiner (SANE) may also be needed for some practice settings.

CORE COMPETENCIES/SKILLS NEEDED
- Ability to work in diverse conditions and deal with emotionally charged issues
- Ability to combine nursing knowledge with investigative and counseling skills
- Ability to collaborate with experts in other disciplines
- Be an advocate for victims
- Coordinate programs in collaboration with medical and law enforcement
- Be able to deal with death and dying

RELATED WEB SITE AND PROFESSIONAL ORGANIZATION
- Forensic Nursing Services (http://www.forensicnursing.org)

70 ■ FRAUD AND ABUSE INVESTIGATOR

BASIC DESCRIPTION
A fraud and abuse investigator investigates health care fraud and abuse charges using such techniques as information technology and statistics to identify outlier practice behaviors. They are employed by government agencies or by independent consulting groups who perform services through contacts with government agencies. This allows investigators to recognize and look more closely at providers who are practicing in an unusual manner. Investigations are often aggressive and involve working with the FBI and US Attorneys to obtain justice. Cases are also reported to local medical and professional boards. The most common types of fraud and abuse are upcoding (e.g., a practitioner billing for a 60-minute office visit when it was only a 20-minute visit); unbundling (e.g., usually dealing with CPT coding, like a blood test being billed under a combined code, then one or more tests from that composite test gets billed individually); charging for services not rendered; and performing unnecessary procedures or tests.

EDUCATIONAL REQUIREMENTS
Registered nurse preparation and an undergraduate degree are the baseline on which to add additional skills, certifications, and expertise. Graduate degree in business is desired.

CORE COMPETENCIES/SKILLS NEEDED
- Computer literacy; cases are often complex with myriad databases requiring an understanding of information technology
- A broad background in nursing with up-to-date clinical knowledge
- Experience and understanding of the health care system
- Law-related areas of study are valuable, as is an in-depth understanding of managed care, risk management, and contracts

- Understanding of annual reports and budgets
- An understanding of statistics is important because current investigative techniques are often computer generated and driven and involve the use of statistics
- Recognition that the cost of fraud is paid by everyone and that health care dollars are finite
- An understanding that money spent on dishonest reimbursement reduces the amount of money available for preventative and other appropriate care

RELATED WEB SITE AND PROFESSIONAL ORGANIZATION

- Electronic Data Systems (http://www.eds.com/health_care/medicaid/hc_medicaid_white_paper_dec.shtml)

71 ■ GASTROENTEROLOGY NURSE

BASIC DESCRIPTION
Gastroenterology nursing is a specialty practice area in which nurses provide care to patients with known or suspected gastrointestinal problems and who are undergoing diagnostic or therapeutic treatment and/or procedures. This area of nursing has expanded because of increased technology and new screening procedures. Practice environments are usually available in endoscopy departments in hospitals, clinics, or physicians' offices, as well as in ambulatory outpatient endoscopy facilities.

EDUCATIONAL REQUIREMENTS
Registered nurse preparation is required. National certification in the specialty is available through the Certifying Board of Gastroenterology Nurses. This board sets the requirements for obtaining and maintaining certification. Certified registered nurses earn the credential Certified Gastroenterology Registered Nurse. Generally, nurses have experience in medical–surgical nursing prior to electing to specialize.

CORE COMPETENCIES/SKILLS NEEDED
- Technical competency
- Maturity
- Empathy
- Knowledge of pathophysiology of gastrointestinal system
- Physical assessment and screening skills
- Case management skills

RELATED WEB SITES AND PROFESSIONAL ORGANIZATIONS
- Society of Gastroenterology Nurses and Associates, Inc. (www.sgna.org)
- Gastroenterology Nursing (www.gastroenterologynursing.com)
- Board of Certification for Gastroenterology Nurses, Inc. (www.abcgn.org)

72 ■ GENERAL PRACTICE NURSE ANESTHETIST

BASIC DESCRIPTION

Nurse anesthetists are responsible for inducing anesthesia, maintaining it at the required levels, and supporting life functions while anesthesia is being administered. Nurse anesthetists administer all types of anesthesia and may perform general, local, and regional anesthesia procedures to pediatric, adult, and geriatric patients, using invasive monitoring techniques when necessary. These nurses practice as part of a highly skilled interdisciplinary team. A variety of practice settings exist including

- Emergency rooms
- Operating rooms
- Physicians' offices
- Plastic surgery practices
- Dental practices
- Orthopedic practices

EDUCATIONAL REQUIREMENTS

Registered nurse (RN) preparation with Certified Registered Nurse Anesthetist certification is required; Master of Science in Nursing is preferred. To enter a nurse anesthetist program, one must possess an active RN license and a baccalaureate degree (may or may not be in nursing). The person must also fulfill certain prerequisites before applying, which vary according to institution. The applicant must also possess a minimum of 1 year of critical care experience as an RN.

CORE COMPETENCIES/SKILLS NEEDED

- Assessment skills and a constant awareness of what is going on at all times
- Skill in history taking and physical assessment
- Patient education skills

- Ability to recognize and take appropriate corrective action (including consulting with anesthesiologist) for abnormal patient responses
- Excellent observation skills
- Ability to provide resuscitative care until the patient has regained control of vital functions
- Skill in administering spinal, epidural, auxiliary, and field blocks

RELATED WEB SITES AND PROFESSIONAL ORGANIZATIONS

- American Association of Nurse Anesthetists (www.aana.com)
- Council on Certification of Nurse Anesthetists

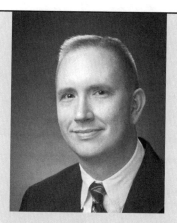

Profile:
CHRISTOPHER REINHART
Nurse Anesthetist

1. What is your educational background in nursing (and other areas) and what formal credentials do you hold?

I became a registered nurse (RN) through a 2-year diploma program. I then earned a Bachelor of Science in Nursing (BSN), Master of Science in Nursing (MSN) with a major in Nurse Anesthesia, and then the professional doctorate, the Doctorate of Nursing Practice (DNP).

I maintain certifications in Advanced Cardiac Life Support, Pediatric Advanced Life Support, Neonatal Resuscitation Program, Basic Cardiac Life Support, and paramedic licensure (EMT-P).

2. How did you first become interested in the career that you are currently in?

I first became intrigued in nurse anesthesia after meeting a Certified Registered Nurse Anesthetist (CRNA) while I was a nursing student completing my clinicals in the operating room. After working in critical care areas for 5 years as a RN, I wanted additional responsibility in a different type of critical care environment. I researched the nurse anesthesia profession, then I interviewed and shadowed several CRNAs before choosing to enter a nurse anesthetist program.

3. What are the most rewarding aspects of your career?

Rewarding aspects of my career include having the ability to calm nervous patients and tend to their needs while they are under anesthesia; being able to relieve a laboring mother's pain shortly after

Continued

101

Profile: CHRISTOPHER REINHART Continued

meeting her through patient education and then administration of a spinal or labor epidural; and obtaining respect from my colleagues.

I love doing the job I do, and the results of my work are frequently instantaneous. It is not uncommon to be called to emergency situations anywhere in the hospital to manage an airway or insert a breathing tube to help save a patient's life.

4. What advice would you give to someone contemplating the same career path in nursing?

If you enjoy working as a RN in the intensive care unit (ICU) or other critical care areas, a career as a CRNA may be for you! The job of a CRNA can be routine at times; however, a patient's condition can deteriorate at a moment's notice requiring critical thinking and rapid interventions from the CRNA.

Admission into CRNA programs is very competitive. Strive to get the highest GPA possible in your undergraduate preparations. Keep in mind, many hospitals have tuition reimbursement programs for RNs working toward a BSN or MSN. Working in an adult ICU at a larger hospital with high acuity patients can increase your experience as a RN and improve your chances of getting into a CRNA program. (Some programs accept students from other critical care backgrounds and from small and midsized hospitals as well.) Most CRNA programs currently range from 26 to 30 months of full-time training. The option to train part-time does not typically exist. You will have minimal to no time to work as a RN while you are in CRNA training. Therefore, you need to be financially prepared before starting a CRNA program. As CRNA programs continue to transition from the master's degree to the doctorate degree level, training time may be extended.

For additional information, visit the American Association of Nurse Anesthetists Web site at www.aana.com, and shadow a CRNA.

73 ■ GENETICS COUNSELOR

BASIC DESCRIPTION
Genetic counselors are nurses or health professionals with specialized graduate degrees and experience in the areas of genetics and counseling. Most enter the field from a variety of disciplines, including biology, genetics, nursing, psychology, public health, and social work. Genetic counselors frequently speak to clients about complex scientific and emotional topics. They work as members of a health care team providing information and support to families who have members with birth defects or genetic disorders and to families who may be at risk for a variety of inherited conditions. Genetic counselors investigate the problem present in the family, interpret information about the disorder, analyze inheritance patterns and risks of recurrence, review available options with the family, serve as patient advocates, and engage in research activities.

EDUCATIONAL REQUIREMENTS
Educational requirements for the nurse would be a master's degree or PhD with advanced education in genetics such as that offered through the National Institutes of Health. The American Board of Genetic Counseling (ABGC) certifies genetic counselors and accredits genetic counseling training programs. Certification in genetic counseling is available by the ABGC. Requirements include documentation of the following: a graduate degree in genetic counseling; clinical experience in an ABGC-approved training site or sites; a log book of 50 supervised cases; and successful completion of both the general and specialty certification examination. Certification as advance practice or clinical nurse in genetics is also available from the Advanced Practice Nurse in Genetics Genetic Nursing Credentialing Commission, Inc.

CORE COMPETENCIES/SKILLS NEEDED
- Knowledge of inherited diseases and the ability to counsel parents and families regarding genetic possibilities
- Critical thinking skills

- Collaborative team practice skills
- Deep sensitivity to patient and family concerns
- Listening skills
- Maturity

RELATED WEB SITES AND PROFESSIONAL ORGANIZATIONS

- National Society of Genetic Counselors, Inc. (www.nsgc.org)
- Online Journal of Genetic Counseling (www.kluweronline.com/issn/1059-7700)
- The American Board of Genetic Counseling, Inc. (www.faseb.org/genetics/abgc/abgcmenu.htm)
- Advance Practice Nurse in Genetics Genetic Nursing Credentialing Commission, Inc. (www.geneticnurse.org)

74 ■ GERIATRIC NURSE PRACTITIONER

BASIC DESCRIPTION
Geriatric nurse practitioners provide primary and acute care to older persons. They work in hospitals, nursing homes, clinics, home care agencies, senior citizen centers, and in wellness programs in the community.

EDUCATIONAL REQUIREMENTS
Registered nurse preparation and a graduate degree from a gerontological nurse practitioner program are required. Certification from American Nurses Credentialing Center is available. Certification as a gerontology clinical nurse specialist, another advanced nursing practice role, is available from the American Nurses Credentialing Center.

CORE COMPETENCIES/SKILLS NEEDED
- Skills in development and implementation of treatment plans for chronic illness
- Ability to provide support, education, and counseling for families
- Understanding of the special needs of the elderly and the process of aging
- Skills in coordination of care

RELATED WEB SITES AND PROFESSIONAL ORGANIZATIONS
- National Association of Professional Geriatric Care Managers (www.caremanager.org/)
- National Gerontological Nursing Association (www.ngna.org)
- American Academy of Nurse Practitioners (www.aanp.org)
- American College of Nurse Practitioners (www.nurse.org/acnp)
- American Nurses Credentialing Center (www.nursecredentialing. org)

75 ■ GEROPSYCHIATRIC NURSE

BASIC DESCRIPTION

The geropsychiatric nurse is someone who specializes in caring for older adults with a diagnosis of depression, dementia, and other mental health disorders. They are employed in various health care settings such as home care, ambulatory care settings, and acute care facilities.

EDUCATIONAL REQUIREMENTS

Registered nurse license and Bachelor of Science in Nursing are highly preferred; an additional education and training and previous experience in mental health or gerontology are usually required for the position; Basic Life Support certification is also required.

CORE COMPETENCIES/SKILLS NEEDED

- Knowledge of physiological changes, common pathophysiological disorders, unique needs, psychopharmacology, and behavioral management among older adults
- Excellent communication and assessment skills
- Knowledge of evidence-based information related to the care of older adults who have dementia and other mental health disorders
- Strong analytical and critical thinking skills

RELATED WEB SITE AND PROFESSIONAL ORGANIZATION

- Hartford Institute for Geriatric Nursing (http://hartfordign.org/education/geropsych_nursing_comp/)

76 ■ HEALTH CARE SURVEYOR

BASIC DESCRIPTION

A health care surveyor nurse is responsible for ensuring that health care providers and health care agencies meet state and federal statutes and regulations. Responsibilities may include surveying health care agencies, investigating complaints against health care professionals, health care agencies, auditing Medicaid claims, and participating in disaster or health care emergencies.

EDUCATIONAL REQUIREMENTS

A Bachelor of Science in Nursing is required; master's degree is preferred; current registered nurse license and successful completion of prerequisite training course within the first year of employment are required.

CORE COMPETENCIES/SKILLS NEEDED

- Requires travel, and flexibility with time
- Extensive knowledge of state and federal health care standards and regulations
- Basic computer skills
- Excellent written and interpersonal communication skills
- Ability to work with members of the health care team

RELATED WEB SITE AND PROFESSIONAL ORGANIZATION

- State Department of Health

77 ■ HEALTH AND SAFETY MANAGER

BASIC DESCRIPTION

In the role of an administrator, a health and safety manager nurse develops system-wide programs to ensure the delivery of safe and quality care in a health care organization. Using her/his clinical and analytical skills, he/she serves as a consultant and a key management personnel to administrators in interpreting and analyzing clinical and administrative data.

EDUCATIONAL REQUIREMENTS

Registered nurse preparation and master's degree or higher in nursing or a health-related field are required.

CORE COMPETENCIES/SKILLS NEEDED

- At least 5 years of leadership and managerial experience in health care
- Strong communication and interpersonal skills
- Knowledge of risk management and quality improvement principles, Joint Commission regulations, and safety principles
- Strong skills in data management

RELATED WEB SITE AND PROFESSIONAL ORGANIZATION

- American Organization of Nurse Executives (http://www.aone.org/)

78 ■ HEALTH CENTER NURSE

BASIC DESCRIPTION

The health center nurse provides a comprehensive range of services to individuals and families that range from conducting a health history and health screening; assisting physicians and other health care providers with procedures; administering treatments, immunizations, and medications per physician's order; and maintaining charts and ensuring proper documentation. They may also be required to take an active role in cases of public health emergency. A health center nurse works in ambulatory centers, home care agencies, or public health organizations.

EDUCATIONAL REQUIREMENTS

A registered nurse license is required; Basic Life Support certification is required.

CORE COMPETENCIES/SKILLS NEEDED

- Strong assessment and analytical skills
- Strong computer and documentation skills
- Flexibility, assertiveness, and creativity
- Excellent interpersonal and communication skills
- Knowledge of public health laws
- Ability to work with other members of the health care team
- May also assume managerial responsibilities if working in ambulatory centers

RELATED WEB SITE AND PROFESSIONAL ORGANIZATION

- National Association of Community Health Centers (www.nachc.org)

79 ▪ HEALTH COACH

BASIC DESCRIPTION

Health coaches are primarily registered nurses (RNs), but also respiratory therapists and dieticians, who work with patients around the clock offering services completely by telephone. They provide state-of-the-art health information and a calming voice when a patient is having a crisis or is in pain or indecision, and provide tips on self-care. Health coaches stay in contact with their patients and provide information and support until the patient begins to feel better and gain confidence. Coaches have more time with patients to provide them with new tools and more support, thereby helping them understand their conditions better and navigate their way through the health care system. Patients will sometimes reveal things over the phone that they would not say in person, fostering deep interactions with their health coach. A large part of health coaching is encouraging patients to become actively involved in their own health and to work with their health care providers in making critical health decisions. Patients are also encouraged to manage their health conditions in ways that reflect the patients' personal values and preferences. Health coaches generally work for independent companies; they also may be independent consultants.

EDUCATIONAL REQUIREMENTS

RN preparation is required.

CORE COMPETENCIES/SKILLS NEEDED

- Excellent listening and interpersonal skills based on the fact that all services are telephone based

- Extensive clinical knowledge
- Knowledge of health promotion, illness prevention, and treatment
- Counseling skills

RELATED WEB SITES AND PROFESSIONAL ORGANIZATIONS

- Health Coach Training Programs and Certification (www.worldhealthandhealing.com/)
- WebMD (www.webmd.com)

BASIC DESCRIPTION

Nurse lobbyists lobby for issues, particularly those related to health care legislation or health policy. A health policy analyst collects data and conducts background research, synthesizes research findings, and reports this information in verbal or written formats, usually on a particular project that serves the client's needs. Because of the analyst's knowledge of health and health care, the data and background documents are framed to convey information about the broad determinants of health and the impact of the data on policy change. A successful lobbyist must perform detailed policy analysis, understand the complex processes of policy making, establish strong relationships with decision makers, create a trustworthy and approachable reputation, and know the culture of the lawmakers and utilize congruent political strategies. Health policy analysts and lobbyists may be independent consultants or may be employed by professional organizations. Health policy analysts may be employed by government agencies (e.g., state or city health departments).

EDUCATIONAL REQUIREMENTS

Registered nurse preparation is required; Master of Science in Nursing and Master of Public Health or equivalent are desired.

CORE COMPETENCIES/SKILLS NEEDED

- Legislative background
- Analytical skills in public health and health care issues
- Knowledge of political and legislative processes
- Appropriate research skills to seek a variety of data sources, and to prioritize among the data sources for accuracy and bias
- Excellent and accurate attention to detail is required in all written and verbal communication
- Ability to effectively prioritize project tasks and schedules

■ Broad knowledge of key processes related to legislation, regulation, and politics on the local, state, and legislative levels
■ Ability to extract and summarize large amounts of data and evidence to support health policies

RELATED WEB SITES AND PROFESSIONAL ORGANIZATIONS

■ State of CT ethics commission lobbyist electronic filing (www.lims.state.CT.us/public/eth4b.asp)
■ North Carolina Nurses Association (www.ncnurses.org/leg_info.htm)

81 ■ HEALTH CARE DISPUTE ANALYST

BASIC DESCRIPTION

Employed in a health care management organization, a health care dispute analyst nurse reviews appeals and billing disputes to ensure that medical claims have been paid correctly. She/he makes recommendations for approval or denial of claims based on her assessment and analysis.

EDUCATIONAL REQUIREMENTS

Registered nurse preparation is required; Bachelor of Science in Nursing is highly preferred. Certification in Managed Care Nursing is available from the American Board of Managed Care Nursing.

CORE COMPETENCIES/SKILLS NEEDED

- Understanding of health care payment and reimbursement process
- Knowledge of ICD-9 codes and experience with CPT-4 coding
- Strong computer skills and documentation skills
- Strong organizational skills and ability to work efficiently with multiple documents and data

RELATED WEB SITES AND PROFESSIONAL ORGANIZATIONS

- Aetna Health Organization (http://www.aetna.com/healthcare-professionals/policies-guidelines/dispute_process.html)
- Centers for Medicare and Medicaid Services (http://www.cms.gov/QualityImprovementOrgs/01_Overview.asp)
- American Board of Managed Care Nursing (www.abmcn.org)

82 ■ HERBALIST

BASIC DESCRIPTION
The herbalist nurse assists patients in the proper and safe use of herbal medicine in the patient medical care regimen especially when used with pharmaceutical agents. Herbalist registered nurses (RNs) combine their knowledge of nursing and herbal medicine to design individualized treatment plans.

EDUCATIONAL REQUIREMENTS
RN preparation and advanced education on herbal medicine are required.

CORE COMPETENCIES/SKILLS NEEDED
- Advanced knowledge of herbal medicine
- Strong knowledge on pharmacokinetics and pharmacodynamics
- Excellent interpersonal and communication skills

RELATED WEB SITES AND PROFESSIONAL ORGANIZATIONS
- Tai Sophia Institute (http://www.tai.edu/)
- American Herbal Products Association (http://www.ahpa.org/)
- American Botanical Council (http://abc.herbalgram.org/site/PageServer?pagename=Homepage)
- American Herbalist Guild (http://www.americanherbalistguild.com)

83 ■ HISTORIAN

BASIC DESCRIPTION
The nurse historian documents and identifies the dilemmas with which nursing has struggled throughout time. History provides current nurses with the same intellectual and political tools that determined nursing pioneers applied to shape nursing values and beliefs to the social context of their times. Nursing history includes the study of labor history, gender studies, oral and social history, anthropology, and the social sciences. Such study exposes nursing students, practitioners, faculty, and administrators to the helpfulness of using history to understand the evolution of the profession. It provides a historical perspective to debates on health policy, encourages reflective practice among nursing professionals, and provides the historical legacy of the profession. Nurse historians are most often employed by academic institutions and the historical research is completed as part of their scholarship.

EDUCATIONAL REQUIREMENTS
PhD is required to do the historical research and to hold a university faculty position as a nurse historian.

CORE COMPETENCIES/SKILLS NEEDED
- Interest in doing historical research and teaching
- Ability to attend to details
- Skills in historical research methods

RELATED WEB SITES AND PROFESSIONAL ORGANIZATIONS
- American Association for the History of Nursing, Inc. (www.aahn.org)
- American Nurses Association Hall of Fame (www.ana.org/hof/index.htm#about)

84 ■ HIV/AIDS SPECIALIST

BASIC DESCRIPTION

An HIV/AIDS specialist is a nurse who works primarily with patients inflicted with HIV/AIDS. HIV/AIDS specialists may work in acute care facilities, long-term care facilities, home care, and hospice.

EDUCATIONAL REQUIREMENTS

Registered nurse (RN) preparation is required. Palliative care certification is available, but not always required for job placement; certification by *Association of Nurses in AIDS Care* or HIV/AIDS Nursing Certification Board is available as AIDS Certified RN or Advance AIDS Certified RN.

CORE COMPETENCIES/SKILLS NEEDED

- Expertise in caring for those who have HIV/AIDS
- Extensive knowledge of HIV/AIDS disease process
- Knowledge of death, dying, and grieving process
- Skills to provide counseling to families of those inflicted with HIV/AIDS
- Ability to care, manage, and teach those inflicted
- Assessment skills for pain and pain management techniques
- Knowledge and understanding of the ethical issues that arise at the end of life

RELATED WEB SITES AND PROFESSIONAL ORGANIZATIONS

- Association of Nurses in AIDS Care (www.anacnet.org)
- World Home Care and Hospice Organization (www.whho.org)
- HIV/AIDS Nursing Certification Board (www.handcb.org)

85 ■ HOLISTIC HEALTH NURSE

BASIC DESCRIPTION

Holistic nursing involves all aspects of wellness and healing of a holistic nature, with holism defined as the mind-body-spirit connection. Holistic nurses treat the whole person, not just a disease or symptom. Working as a holistic nurse is a chance to be a part of a growing specialty, but because the field is new, some skepticism still exists. Opportunities for employment exist in health care facilities, holistic health and wellness centers, spas and health clubs, private practices, and pain management centers.

EDUCATIONAL REQUIREMENTS

Registered nurse preparation is required. Certification in holistic nursing is available from the American Holistic Nurses' Certification Corporation.

CORE COMPETENCIES/SKILLS NEEDED

- Interest in—and commitment to focus on—wellness, healing, and illness prevention from a more spiritual and natural perspective
- Commitment to a holistic philosophy
- Knowledge of complementary and alternative therapies
- Openness to go beyond the conventions of traditional medicine and health care

RELATED WEB SITES AND PROFESSIONAL ORGANIZATIONS

- American Holistic Nurses' Association (www.ahna.org)
- The RN Reiki Connection (http://member.aol.com/KarunaRN/)
- American Holistic Nurses' Certification Corporation (www.ahncc.org)

86 ■ HOME HEALTH CARE NURSE PRACTITIONER

BASIC DESCRIPTION
Home health care nurse practitioners provide home-based care to chronically ill patients across age groups. They conduct assessment, diagnose disease conditions, order and provide treatment, and evaluate patient care. They also provide referral services if necessary. They work with members of the health care and maintain close communication with patients and caregivers.

EDUCATIONAL REQUIREMENTS
Registered nurse preparation, a master's degree and Nurse Practitioner certification are required.

CORE COMPETENCIES/SKILLS NEEDED
- Excellent assessment and analytical skills
- Ability to work independently
- Knowledge of home health care regulations and reimbursement
- Excellent organizational, leadership, and communication skills
- Knowledge of regulations on advance directives and end-of-life care

RELATED WEB SITES AND PROFESSIONAL ORGANIZATIONS
- American College of Nurse Practitioners (http://www.acnpweb. org/i4a/pages/index.cfm?pageid=1)
- National Association for Home Care and Hospice (http://www.nahc.org/)
- Visiting Nurse Service of New York (http://www.vnsny.org/our-services/)

87 ■ HOME HEALTH NURSE

BASIC DESCRIPTION

A home health nurse provides nursing care and support to individuals and families in their own homes, assisted living facilities, or nursing homes. This care may be provided before or after acute and long-term illness. Home health nurses may be prepared as generalists for care of all patients or may be specialists (e.g., oncology or geriatric nurses). Home health nurses provide direct patient care in contrast to public or community health nurses whose focus is population based.

EDUCATIONAL REQUIREMENTS

Registered nurse preparation is required.

CORE COMPETENCIES/SKILLS NEEDED

- Ability to function independently at an optimal level
- Excellent communication and bedside manner with patients and their families
- The ability to perceive the patient's needs in relation to the home environment
- The ability to conform and adapt traditional nursing care to the home environment
- Knowledge of many cultures and openness to work with people from a wide variety of cultures
- Excellent assessment skills
- Autonomy and flexibility

RELATED WEB SITES AND PROFESSIONAL ORGANIZATIONS

- National Association for Home Care (www.nahc.org)
- Home Healthcare Nurses Association (www.nahc.org/HHNA)
- Visiting Nurse Associations of America (www.vnaa.org)

88 ■ HOSPICE AND PALLIATIVE CARE NURSE

BASIC DESCRIPTION

Hospice/palliative care nurses work with people who have a terminal illness and are predicted to die within 6 months. Hospice/palliative care can take place in a hospice facility, but approximately 90% receive care at home or other residential care institutions. Nurses who work with dying patients and their loved ones must be able to manage dealing with death on a daily basis; the stress of the work requires maturity.

EDUCATIONAL REQUIREMENTS

Registered nurse preparation is required. Usually 1 to 2 years of experience in home care and oncology is recommended before entering this specialty. Certification in various roles is available in this specialty (CHPN) through the National Board for Certification of Hospice and Palliative Nurses.

CORE COMPETENCIES/SKILLS NEEDED

- Attention to the psychological, spiritual, physical, and social aspects of care as related to the patient's quality of life
- Skill in using resources found within the home or other residential site to provide end-of-life nursing care
- Ability to provide stress relief for dying patients and their families
- Skill in relieving multiple physical symptoms such as pain, dyspnea, fatigue, anorexia, and delirium
- Skill in helping patients deal with emotional symptoms such as depression, anxiety, and fear associated with facing impending death
- Collaboration with other members of the interdisciplinary team to help relieve patient suffering

RELATED WEB SITES AND PROFESSIONAL ORGANIZATIONS

- Hospice and Palliative Nurses Association (www.hpna.org)
- Hospice Association of America (www.hospice-america.org)
- World Home Care and Hospice Organization (www.whho.org)
- End-of-Life Nursing Education Consortium (www.aacn.nche. edu/elnec)
- National Board for Certification of Hospice and Palliative Nurses (www.nbchpn.org)

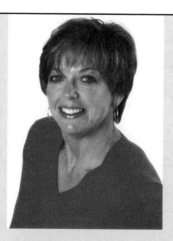

Profile:
MALENE DAVIS
Hospice Nurse

1. What is your educational background in nursing (and other areas) and what formal credentials do you hold?

I am a registered nurse and hold a bachelor's of science degree, a master's of science degree in nursing, and an MBA. I am also a Certified Hospice and Palliative Nurse.

2. How did you first become interested in the career that you are currently in?

I began as a nurse in oncology and was initially very interested in the science behind treating cancer and serious diseases. Over time, as I watched patients experience the pain and difficult symptoms associated with a lot of advanced medical treatments, I found that it was critical to provide holistic care, by not only offering compassion, but by offering pain relief and symptom management.

This experience coupled with my personal encounter with hospice with my grandmother who just wanted to "go home" compelled me to found the nonprofit Hospice Care Corporation in Arthurdale, WV, in 1988, which has become the largest hospice program in the state. I started it from the ground up! My next personal encounter was in 1998 when my beloved father was dying.

Continued

Profile: MALENE DAVIS Continued

3. What are the most rewarding aspects of your career?

I have been actively promoting palliative and hospice care for most of my career. The most rewarding aspect of this has been leading a movement that, over time, will enhance the lives of thousands of patients and families who are coping with advanced illnesses. As our nation's aging population surges, the need for coordinated, holistic care will become that much more relevant. I can't think of a better job to have than to promote this type of care so that Americans from coast-to-coast have dignity and comfort in the face of serious illness.

4. What advice would you give to someone contemplating the same career path in nursing?

Nursing is, first and foremost, about providing excellent clinical care and compassion to people who are sick. If you have a desire to do that and to do more than that, as I have done, opportunities abound. This is particularly true as our country reexamines the current health care system and looks for better ways to improve medical care. The simple truth is we need good nurses. They are the backbone of our health system. If you feel this is your calling, I encourage you to pursue nursing with verve and vigor. Your efforts will pay off!

89 ■ IN VITRO FERTILIZATION NURSE

BASIC DESCRIPTION

Acting as coaches, guides, and support, in vitro fertilization (IVF) nurses assist patients in streamlining the processes involved in IVF. They coordinate diagnostic and treatment schedules and educate patients and their partners about medication administration, testing preparation, and specimen collection.

EDUCATIONAL REQUIREMENTS

A registered nurse license required.

CORE COMPETENCIES/SKILLS NEEDED
- Knowledge of Food and Drug Administration regulations regarding fertility treatments
- Excellent organization and communication skills
- Knowledge of diagnostic procedures and treatments and latest evidence-based information related to fertility and fertility treatment

RELATED WEB SITES AND PROFESSIONAL ORGANIZATIONS
- Society for Reproductive Endocrinology and Infertility (www.socrei.org)
- Resolve: The National Infertility Association (www.resolve.org)
- Society for Assisted Reproductive Technologies (www.sart.org)

90 ■ INFECTION CONTROL NURSE

BASIC DESCRIPTION
An infection control nurse is a nurse who specializes in identifying, controlling, and preventing outbreaks of infection in health care settings and the community. These nurses establish and implement guidelines directed toward the prevention, detection, and control of infectious processes. Activities include the collection and analysis of infection control data; the planning, implementation, and evaluation of infection prevention and control measures; the education of individuals about infection risk, prevention, and control; the development and revision of infection control policies and procedures; the investigation of suspected outbreaks of infection; and the provision of consultation on infection risk assessment, prevention, and control strategies. Practice areas include long-term care facilities, community or regional hospitals, nonacute inpatient institutions, industry, private and public settings, nursing homes, and mental health facilities.

EDUCATIONAL REQUIREMENTS
Registered nurse preparation and Bachelor of Science in Nursing are required; documented educational programs related to epidemiology, sterilization, sanitation, disinfection, patient care practice, and adult education principles are a requirement. Certification as an infection control practitioner is preferred and is available from the Certification Board of Infection Control and Epidemiology, Inc. Master of Science in Nursing or Master of Public Health may be required.

CORE COMPETENCIES/SKILLS NEEDED
- Ability to diagnose HIV/AIDS, tuberculosis, scabies, nosocomial infections, and other infectious diseases
- Knowledge of prevention of infectious diseases

- Knowledge and expertise in microbiology, epidemiology, statistics, sterilization and disinfection, infectious diseases, and antibiotic usage
- Consultative and teaching skills
- Knowledge of the multitude of federal and organizational mandates

RELATED WEB SITES AND PROFESSIONAL ORGANIZATIONS
- Centers for Disease Control and Prevention (www.cdc.gov)
- Association for Professionals in Infection Control and Epidemiology, Inc. (www.apic.org)
- Certification Board of Infection Control and Epidemiology, Inc. (www.cbic.org)

91 ■ INFECTIOUS DISEASE NURSE PRACTITIONER

BASIC DESCRIPTION
Infectious disease nurse practitioners work across all health care settings to prevent, manage, and treat infectious diseases. They can serve as educators, health policy makers and advocates, direct care providers, or researchers.

EDUCATIONAL REQUIREMENTS
Registered nurse preparation, master's degree, and certification in infection control are required.

CORE COMPETENCIES/SKILLS NEEDED
- Knowledge of epidemiology and statistics
- Knowledge of health policy impacting infection control and risk assessment
- Excellent verbal and written communication skills
- Strong computer and interpersonal skills
- Ability to work in a team

RELATED WEB SITES AND PROFESSIONAL ORGANIZATIONS
- Certification Board of Infection Control (www.cbic.org)
- Association of Professionals in Infection Control (www.apic.org)
- Center for Disease Control and Prevention (www.cdc.gov)

92 ■ INFORMATICS SPECIALIST

BASIC DESCRIPTION
Informatics nursing is the integration of nursing and its information management with information processing and communication technology to support the health of people worldwide. Nursing informatics is the specialty that integrates science, computer science, and information science in identifying, collecting, processing, and managing data and information to support nursing practice, administration, research, and the expansion of nursing knowledge. Nursing informatics is considered by many executives as a way to improve quality of care and reduce excess expenditures. Informatics nurses work in a variety of settings such as hospitals, clinics, educational settings, and private consulting firms.

EDUCATIONAL REQUIREMENTS
Bachelor of Science in Nursing is required. Masters degree in nursing informatics preferred. Credentialing is available through the American Nurses Credentialing Center.

CORE COMPETENCIES/SKILLS NEEDED
- Ability to conduct major analyses of information
- Skill in developing data analysis systems and methodologies
- Consultation skills regarding the use of technology
- Marketing skills
- Skill in developing and disseminating reports to staff about cost and other trends in health care
- Ability to use various resources to analyze and interpret variances and make comparisons with national and regional benchmarks
- Ability to manage multiple priorities
- Ability to work independently

RELATED WEB SITES AND PROFESSIONAL ORGANIZATIONS
- American Medical Informatics Association: Nursing Informatics Working Group (www.amia-niwg.org)
- American Nurses Credentialing Center (www.nursingworld.org)
- American Nursing Informatics Association (www.ania.org)

93 ■ INFUSION THERAPY NURSE

BASIC DESCRIPTION

An infusion nurse has expertise in the field of infusion therapy. The infusion nurse's role is to perform intravenous therapy as well as patient education regarding the task being performed. There are opportunities for infusion therapy nurses to work in hospitals, home care, and various alternative settings such as hospice or long-term care facilities.

EDUCATIONAL REQUIREMENTS

Registered nurse preparation is required. Certification is available from the Infusion Nurses Certification Corporation.

CORE COMPETENCIES/SKILLS NEEDED

- Skill in venipuncture
- Knowledge of ways to insure quality care to patients
- Knowledge of nosocomial infection rates and prevention
- Good interpersonal skills

RELATED WEB SITES AND PROFESSIONAL ORGANIZATIONS

- Infusion Nurses Society (www.ins1.org)
- Infusion Nurses Certification Corporation (www.incc1.org)

94 ■ INTAKE NURSE

BASIC DESCRIPTION

Intake registered nurses are sometimes the first health care professionals that patients meet in the acute care setting. Their responsibilities may include conducting an initial assessment and obtaining nursing history for newly admitted patients. Aside from providing patients with an overview of the unit, they may also determine the types and intensity of services that patients will receive in a particular unit.

EDUCATIONAL REQUIREMENTS

In hospitals that have specific job description for this role, a Bachelor of Science in Nursing is highly preferred and several years of acute care experience is a requirement.

CORE COMPETENCIES/SKILLS NEEDED
- Good assessment, triage, and interview skills
- Excellent communication skills and knowledge of specific services in the hospital
- Excellent organization skills and basic computer skills
- Ability to work in a fast-paced environment

RELATED WEB SITE AND PROFESSIONAL ORGANIZATION
- None

95 ■ INTERNATIONAL HEALTH NURSE

BASIC DESCRIPTION
An international health nurse may work on a wide range of global health issues in a number of settings. They may be employed by government agencies (e.g., the United Nations, the World Health Organization, or nongovernmental organizations). They also could be independent consultants. The topics of importance to global nursing include the increasing disparity in access to health care; the growing population of the poor (more than one billion people do not have access to basic health and social care, regardless of availability); the rapid environmental changes and degradation of the environment; economic recession and crises in parts of the world that affect the financing of health care; the inability of technology to face epidemics and deadly threats from diseases such as HIV/AIDS, malaria, and tuberculosis; the growing crises and emergencies such as internal conflicts, civil wars, and natural disasters that affect the health delivery systems and access to care.

International health nurses are committed to care for all persons across the life cycle—pregnant women, infants, children, adolescents, adults, and the elderly—and especially vulnerable groups—the poor, refugees and displaced persons, street children, and the homeless.

In setting the future directions for global health policy, nursing and midwifery are key elements. As nurses and midwives already constitute up to 80% of the qualified health workforce in most national health systems, they represent a potentially powerful force for bringing about the necessary changes to meet the needs of health for all in the 21st century. Their contribution to health services covers the whole spectrum of health care, promotion and prevention, as well as health research, planning, implementation, and innovation.

EDUCATIONAL REQUIREMENTS
Registered nurse licensure is required; graduate preparation in nursing or public health is desirable.

CORE COMPETENCIES/SKILLS NEEDED

- Knowledge of major global health risks such as HIV/AIDS, tuberculosis, smoking, and environmental hazards
- Knowledge of epidemiology
- Skills in community mobilization for integrated health development
- Immunization knowledge and skills
- Leadership skills
- Skills in preparing nurses to be ready for emergencies and crisis situations
- Disaster planning and intervention skills
- Ability to enhance team building and leadership abilities of nurses as health care providers and planners
- Public health knowledge
- Skill in demonstrating cost-effective care through primary health care and the critical role of nurses in the health care team

RELATED WEB SITES AND PROFESSIONAL ORGANIZATIONS

- World Health Organization (www.who.int/homepage/index.en.shtml)
- International Council of Nurses (www.icn.ch/index.html)
- The Transcultural Nursing Society (www.tcns.org)

96 ■ INTERVENTIONAL RADIOLOGY NURSE PRACTITIONER

BASIC DESCRIPTION

The interventional radiology nurse practitioner—a practice role—works in either acute care setting or ambulatory centers caring for the patient undergoing radiologic imaging procedures and radiation oncology treatments. They are responsible for obtaining consents for the procedure, conducting a thorough physical assessment and medical/surgical history, and evaluating patients pre- and post-procedure.

EDUCATIONAL REQUIREMENTS

Registered nurse (RN) preparation, Nurse Practitioner certification, and Basic Life Support and Advanced Cardiac Life Support certifications are required; masters in nursing and several years of acute care experience as an RN preferably in the critical care or emergency nursing are requirements.

CORE COMPETENCIES/SKILLS NEEDED

- Excellent assessment and critical thinking skills
- Excellent technical skills such as placement of peripheral and central venous catheters and thoracotomy catheters.
- Excellent organizational, leadership, and communication skills.

RELATED WEB SITES AND PROFESSIONAL ORGANIZATIONS

- Association for Radiologic and Imaging Nursing (https://www. arinursing.org/membership-information.html)
- Society for Interventional Radiology (http://www.scvir.org/)

97 ■ INVENTOR

BASIC DESCRIPTION
Nurse inventors are those who seek solutions to patient care problems or delivery system problems by creating new devices; often these inventions are patented.

EDUCATIONAL REQUIREMENTS
Registered nurse preparation.

CORE COMPETENCIES/SKILLS NEEDED
- Desire to fix a problem that has arisen
- Desire to improve patient and nursing care
- Creativity
- Risk-taking skills
- Tenacity
- Must be innovative
- Belief in their product

RELATED WEB SITES AND PROFESSIONAL ORGANIZATIONS
- United States Patent and Trademark Office (www.uspto.gov)
- www.healthcareinventions.com

98 ■ LABOR AND DELIVERY NURSE

BASIC DESCRIPTION

A labor and delivery nurse works with mothers during the final stages of pregnancy helping with birthing, monitoring the mother's vital signs, and becoming astute in signs and symptoms of possible complications. They are involved in patient education and addressing the psychosocial needs of mothers after delivery.

EDUCATIONAL REQUIREMENTS

Registered nurse preparation is required.

CORE COMPETENCIES/SKILLS NEEDED

- Excellent interpersonal and communication skills
- Excellent assessment skills to asses progression of labor
- Must provide support for the mother after childbirth and monitor newborn immediately after birth

RELATED WEB SITES AND PROFESSIONAL ORGANIZATIONS

- American Nurses Credentialing Center (http://www.nursecredentialing.org/NurseSpecialties/Perinatal.aspx)
- Perinatal Nursing Institute (http://perinatalnursingfw.org/wordpress/)
- Association of Women's Health, Obstetric, and Neonatal Nurses (http://www.awhonn.org/awhonn/)

99 ■ LABOR AND DELIVERY NURSE ANESTHETIST

BASIC DESCRIPTION
A labor and delivery nurse anesthetist works with mothers during childbirth to minimize and/or relieve pain. The labor and delivery nurse anesthetist is expert at providing pain relief that is safe for both the mother and the baby. Further, the labor and delivery nurse anesthetist educates family members about different types of pain management strategies and assists them to choose the best pain relief strategy and anesthesia during labor.

EDUCATIONAL REQUIREMENTS
Registered nurse preparation and certification as Certified Registered Nurse Anesthetist are required; experience in labor and delivery as a registered nurse is mostly required; certification is offered by the National Board on Certification and Recertification of Nurse Anesthetists.

CORE COMPETENCIES/SKILLS NEEDED
- Sensitivity to the needs of the family
- Advance knowledge of obstetrics
- Excellent communication skills in dealing with members of the obstetrics team

RELATED WEB SITES AND PROFESSIONAL ORGANIZATIONS
- American Association of Nurse Anesthetists (http://www.aana.com/)
- International Federation of Nurse Anesthetists (http://ifna-int. org/ifna/news.php)
- National Board on Certification and Recertification of Nurse Anesthetists (http://www.nbcrna.com/)

100 ■ LACTATION COUNSELOR

BASIC DESCRIPTION

Lactation consultants and breast-feeding counselors work closely together when a mother is experiencing a breast-feeding problem. They assess the mother and baby, take her history, observe the mother and baby while breast-feeding, problem solve, develop a plan of care, work with and report to the mother's and baby's primary care providers, and arrange for follow-up.

EDUCATIONAL REQUIREMENTS

The term "lactation consultant" refers to anyone who is working in the field of lactation, either as a volunteer or as a professional. However, certification to become an International Board Certified Lactation Consultant is considered the gold standard. This exam is held once a year worldwide. Criteria that must be met for certification are bachelor's, master's, or doctoral degree—or 4 years of postsecondary education; a minimum of 2,500 hours of practice as a breast-feeding consultant; and a minimum of education specific to breast-feeding within the 3 years prior to the exam.

CORE COMPETENCIES/SKILLS NEEDED

- Excellent interpersonal skills
- Peer counseling skills
- Excellent knowledge of lactation and women's health

RELATED WEB SITES AND PROFESSIONAL ORGANIZATIONS

- International Lactation Consultant Association (www.ilca.org)
- La Leche League International (www.lalecheleague.org)
- International Board of Lactation Consultant Examiners (www.iblce.org)

101 ■ LEARNING/DEVELOPMENTAL DISABILITIES NURSE

BASIC DESCRIPTION
The role of a developmental disabilities nurse is to assist clients with mental and physical disabilities to live as normal and productive a life as possible. This might mean assisting clients with manual and recognition skills to enable them to carry out tasks related to maintaining activities of daily living or developing comprehensive plans with specific goals and objectives. Developmental disabilities nurses work in sheltered workshops, group homes, long-term care facilities, and schools.

EDUCATIONAL REQUIREMENTS
Registered nurse (RN) preparation is required; certification eligibility is available to RNs with a minimum of 4,000 hours (2 years full-time equivalent) of developmental disabilities nursing practice within the past 5 years.

CORE COMPETENCIES/SKILLS NEEDED
- Compassion and complete understanding of the person with a disability
- Patience
- Excellent communication skills
- Understanding of chronic long-term disabilities
- Counseling skills for families
- Ability to work with interdisciplinary teams
- Ability to promote positive life experiences
- Ability to provide care for health and social needs
- Ability to understand physical disabilities and psychological/ emotional needs
- Ability to promote positive images of people with disabilities
- Ability to apply clinical and behavioral nursing interventions to meet the special health care needs of the individual

- Ability to act in the capacity of advocate
- Ability to maximize the client's potential by referring to appropriate resources
- Ability to manage care by coordinating services

RELATED WEB SITE AND PROFESSIONAL ORGANIZATION

- Developmental Disabilities Nurses Association (www.ddna.org/)

102 ■ LEGAL CONSULTANT

BASIC DESCRIPTION
Legal nurse consultants (LNCs) are registered nurses (RNs) who use specialized health care knowledge and expertise to consult on medical-related cases. Legal consultants provide a variety of services to attorneys, insurance companies, and hospitals in legal matters where health, illness, or injury are issues, such as personal injury, product liability, medical negligence, toxic torts, workers' compensation, risk management, and fraud and abuse. LNCs assist claims managers with the investigation, evaluation, and management of general and professional liability claims by obtaining, organizing, reviewing, and summarizing pertinent records and documents. They assist in the procurement of expert reviews and evaluation of care, and they provide input into the claims resolution strategy based on evaluations. They support managers with implementation of risk-management activities, all with the objective of controlling or minimizing losses to protect the assets of the corporation. Other responsibilities include drafting litigation documents, conducting medical and legal research, analyzing medical records in depth, and assisting the claims manager with investigation of general and professional liability claims. Employment opportunities are available in law firms, hospitals, insurance companies, government agencies, and consulting firms, as well as in the form of self-employment.

EDUCATIONAL REQUIREMENTS
RN preparation. Certification is available from the American Legal Nurse Consultant Certification Board.

CORE COMPETENCIES/SKILLS NEEDED
- Clinical experience, preferably in a high-risk area
- Statistical background/data management experience preferred
- Liability claims/paralegal experience or educational equivalent also preferred

- Ability to work independently
- Ability to be a self-starter
- Comfortable making decisions
- Excellent reading and writing skills
- Confidence to talk with experts

RELATED WEB SITES AND PROFESSIONAL ORGANIZATIONS

- American Association of Legal Nurse Consultants (www.aalnc.org)
- The American Association of Nurse Attorneys (www.taana.org)
- Medical-Legal Consulting Institute, Inc. (www.legalnurse.com)

103 ■ LEGISLATOR

BASIC DESCRIPTION
A nurse legislator is a nurse who is elected to public office. Nurse politicians serve in a variety of settings such as US Congress, state government, boards of education, and nursing organizations. Given that there are more than 2.4 million nurses in this country, and that 1 in every 17 female voters is a nurse, this represents an important growth area for nursing influence. There are currently two US congresswomen who are nurses: Rep. Lois Capps from California's 22nd district and Rep. Carolyn McCarthy from New York's 4th district.

EDUCATIONAL REQUIREMENTS
Registered nurse preparation is required. Education and/or experience in the area of political action.

CORE COMPETENCIES/SKILLS NEEDED
- Conviction to fight for your beliefs
- Interest in political and social issues
- Ability to be a decision maker
- Leadership ability
- Ability to identify a problem and develop a position and a plan to address the problem
- Ability to identify and articulate health care issues
- Skills in advocating for change
- Collaborating with other members of the political team
- Designing legislation
- Experience in working for reforms in health care, education, and other identified areas of need

RELATED WEB SITES AND PROFESSIONAL ORGANIZATIONS
- American Nurses Association (www.ana.org)
- The US Congress (www.congress.gov)

104 ■ LOBBYIST

BASIC DESCRIPTION
A nurse lobbyist is an advocate for nursing and other health care professions. Through the art of persuasion, sound legislative knowledge, excellent communication skills, and networking they are able to influence legislative decisions that impact the practice of nursing. Large nursing organizations hire either a full-time lobbyist or a part-time consultant to advance their agenda.

EDUCATIONAL REQUIREMENTS
A master's degree is highly preferred.

CORE COMPETENCIES/SKILLS NEEDED
■ Knowledge of state and federal laws that affect health care and political and legislative procedures
■ Knowledge of the American health system
■ Flexibility, professionalism, and excellent verbal and written communication skills

RELATED WEB SITES AND PROFESSIONAL ORGANIZATIONS
■ American Nurses Association RN Action (http://www.rnaction. org/site/PageServer?pagename=nstat_homepage&ct=1)
■ State Nurses Association

105 ■ LONG-TERM CARE ADMINISTRATOR

BASIC DESCRIPTION

A long-term care administrator heads the overall management and operations of a long-term care facility. He/she oversees interdisciplinary departments in the facility that include nursing, medicine, rehabilitation, diet, activities, and environmental services ensuring that resident and family needs, government and regulatory standards, and personnel needs are addressed while maintaining quality and excellent care. Nurses who have long-term care administrative and clinical experience and expertise are well positioned to assume this leadership role in long-term care facilities.

EDUCATIONAL REQUIREMENTS

A master's degree or higher in nursing, health, or business is preferred; licensing and credentialing are available from the National Association of Long Term Care Administrator Boards. Certification is available from the National Association of Directors of Nursing Administration in Long-Term Care.

CORE COMPETENCIES/SKILLS NEEDED

- Strong leadership and management skills
- Knowledge of long-term care state and federal regulations and reimbursement process
- Strong background in Medicare, Medicaid, and third-payer reimbursement regulations

RELATED WEB SITES AND PROFESSIONAL ORGANIZATIONS

- National Association of Long Term Care Administrator Boards (http://www.nabweb.org/nabweb/default.aspx)
- The National Association of Directors of Nursing Administration in Long Term Care (http://www.nadona.org/)

106 ■ LONG-TERM CARE NURSE

BASIC DESCRIPTION

The long-term care nurse works in a long-term care facility with patients with chronic physical and/or mental disorders, who are primarily elderly. Responsible for the day-to-day care of patients, operation of the facility, staff supervision, assessing program quality, program growth and development, and service excellence often are responsibilities of the long-term care nurse. Working in long-term care requires working with patients with challenging diagnoses. Practice settings include nursing homes and skilled nursing facilities.

EDUCATIONAL REQUIREMENTS

Registered nurse preparation is required. Certification as Gerontology Nurse is available from the American Nurses Credentialing Center.

CORE COMPETENCIES/SKILLS NEEDED

- Prior experience with long-term care
- Medical and surgical nursing experience
- Ability to see death as a part of the natural process of life
- Ability to build long-term relationships with patients and their families
- Ability to build teams and mentor others
- Leadership and organizational ability
- Ability to solve staffing difficulties when they arise

RELATED WEB SITES AND PROFESSIONAL ORGANIZATIONS

- American Long Term and Sub Acute Nurses Association (www.alsna.com)
- American Nurses Credentialing Center (www.nursecredentialing. org)

146

107 ■ MASSAGE THERAPY NURSE

BASIC DESCRIPTION
As a specialty, a massage therapist nurse uses a variety of touch therapies and other holistic approaches to facilitate a client's ability for self-healing.

EDUCATIONAL REQUIREMENTS
Registered nurse licensure with 500 hours of postgraduate education and training in massage and body therapies certified by the National Certification Board for Therapeutic Massage and Bodywork (NCBTMB).

CORE COMPETENCIES/SKILLS NEEDED
■ Excellent communication skills
■ Able to adhere to NCBTMB code of ethics and standards of practice
■ Knowledge of anatomy, physiology, kinesiology, pathology, professional standards, ethics, business, and legal practices

RELATED WEB SITES AND PROFESSIONAL ORGANIZATIONS
■ American Massage Therapy Association (http://www.amtamassage.org/index.html)
■ National Certification Board for Therapeutic Massage and Bodywork (http://www.ncbtmb.org/)
■ National Association of Nurse Massage Therapists (http://www.nanmt.org/)
■ United States Medical Massage Association (http://www.americanmedicalmassage.com/)

108 ■ MEDIA CONSULTANT

BASIC DESCRIPTION

Nurses who are media consultants provide behind-the-scenes and up-front consultation for media in order to present accurate and realistic portrayals of health care, patient care, and the professional practice of nursing.

EDUCATIONAL REQUIREMENTS

Registered nurse (RN) preparation but often RNs with advanced degrees and certifications in their specialty fields are preferred.

CORE COMPETENCIES/SKILLS NEEDED

- Knowledge of television, movie, and stage environments
- Ability to work with a wide variety of individuals from producers to actors
- Ability to work with deadlines
- Ability to work in a fast-paced, rapidly changing environment

RELATED WEB SITES AND PROFESSIONAL ORGANIZATIONS

- Registered Nurse Experts, Inc. (www.rnexperts.com)
- Sigma Theta Tau International—media guide

109 ■ MEDICAL RECORDS AUDITOR

BASIC DESCRIPTION
A medical records auditor audits, examines, verifies, adjusts, and corrects medical records and bills to ensure accuracy and consistency. They report discrepancies to personnel and ensure corrective action is taken in a timely manner. They audit physician billing practices against documentation in the medical record to ensure compliance with all federal, state, and third-party billing requirements, rules, and regulations. Medical records auditors go through medical records to make sure everything is in compliance and all the codes match up for billing purposes.

EDUCATIONAL REQUIREMENTS
Registered nurse preparation is required. Many facilities also prefer that the applicant has some college-level business courses or health care experience.

CORE COMPETENCIES/SKILLS NEEDED
- Strong analytical skills and some basic training skills to teach people how to correct problems
- A basic knowledge of diagnostic-related groups and coding
- A broad knowledge of disease processes, findings, courses of treatment, quality assurance, and risk management are essential

RELATED WEB SITES AND PROFESSIONAL ORGANIZATIONS
- National Committee for Quality Assurance (www.ncqa.org/)
- Agency for Healthcare Research and Quality (www.ahrq.gov/)
- National Association for Healthcare Quality (www.nahq.org/)

110 ■ MEDICAL–SURGICAL NURSE

BASIC DESCRIPTION

Medical–surgical nurses are registered nurses (RNs) who specialize in the care of patients admitted with nonsurgical (medical) and surgical conditions. These nurses work to promote health, prevent disease, and help patients cope with illness. They are advocates and health educators for patients, families, and communities. The medical–surgical nurse has an incredibly complex job. The entry-level medical–surgical nurse makes nursing judgments based on scientific knowledge and relies on procedures and standardized care plans. Nursing care is directed toward alleviating physical and psychosocial health problems. Advancing to an intermediate level, the medical–surgical nurse with experience becomes more skilled in developing individual and innovative care plans to meet client needs. With a broader base of experience, a more advanced clinician cares for clients with complex and unpredictable problems. The most common place of employment is the hospital.

EDUCATIONAL REQUIREMENTS

RN preparation and often Master of Science in Nursing preparation are required. Certification is available through the American Nurses Credentialing Center, from the Academy of Medical–Surgical Nurses or from the Master of Science (MS) Nurses Certification Board.

CORE COMPETENCIES/SKILLS NEEDED

- Excellent observation and assessment skills
- Skill in recording symptoms, reactions, and progress
- Skill in administering medical treatments and examinations
- Knowledge of convalescence and rehabilitation requirements for patients
- Skill in developing, planning, implementing, evaluating, documenting, and managing nursing care

- Patient and family education skills
- Ability to help individuals and groups take steps to improve or maintain their health

RELATED WEB SITES AND PROFESSIONAL ORGANIZATIONS

- American Nurses Credentialing Center (www.nursecredentialing. org)
- Academy of Medical–Surgical Nurses (www.medsugrnurse.org)
- MS Nurses International Certification Board (www.ptcny.com)

111 ■ MILITARY NURSE

BASIC DESCRIPTION
Military nurses are those who serve in the military—army, navy, and air force in active duty, reserve, and civilian positions. Military nurses are among the most respected professionals in their field and enjoy many job-related benefits such as sign-on bonuses, housing allowances, and education loan repayment.

EDUCATIONAL REQUIREMENTS
Registered nurses who have Bachelor of Science in Nursing degrees enter as officers; acute care experiences such as critical care or emergency nursing are desired qualities.

CORE COMPETENCIES/SKILLS NEEDED
- U.S. citizenship
- Must meet medical and moral standards outlined by the military
- Must pass a background security check
- Excellent communication skills
- Flexibility and ability to quickly adjust to different locations if deployed

RELATED WEB SITE AND PROFESSIONAL ORGANIZATION
- Information about Military Nursing (www.military-nurse.com)

112 ■ MINIMUM DATA SET NURSE

BASIC DESCRIPTION
Minimum data set (MDS) nurses are long-term care nurses specializing in assessing the needs of long-term care residents. They are responsible for ensuring that MDS assessments are conducted regularly and that care is coordinated among long-term care residents. MDS is a tool that assesses quality of care among long-term care residents and that has a significant influence in payment and reimbursement of skilled nursing care provided.

EDUCATIONAL REQUIREMENTS
Bachelor of Science in Nursing is often required; certification can be obtained from the American Association of Nurse Assessment Coordinators.

CORE COMPETENCIES/SKILLS NEEDED
- Meticulous attention to details
- Knowledge of state and federal long-term care regulatory standards
- Basic computer skills
- Ability to work with interdisciplinary teams
- Significant long-term care experience

RELATED WEB SITE AND PROFESSIONAL ORGANIZATION
- American Association of Nurse Assessment Coordinators (http://www.aanac.org/)

113 ■ MISSIONARY NURSE

BASIC DESCRIPTION
Missionary nurses consider nursing as a calling and they provide nursing and spiritual care to those less fortunate and who may not share their religious belief or orientation. Some belong to a specific religious organization, and they usually work overseas. They assume various roles such as direct caregivers, nursing educators, nursing home administrators, and ambulatory care center directors.

EDUCATIONAL REQUIREMENTS
Registered nurse preparation is required.

CORE COMPETENCIES/SKILLS NEEDED
- Sensitivity to the needs of the less fortunate
- Ability to work and live overseas for an extended period
- Ability to speak other languages
- Strong interpersonal and communication skills
- Excellent clinical skills

RELATED WEB SITES AND PROFESSIONAL ORGANIZATIONS
- Medical Missionaries of Mary (http://www.medicalmissionariesofmary.com/)
- Evangemed (http://www.evangemed.org/)

114 ■ MOTHER/BABY NURSE

BASIC DESCRIPTION

Mother/baby nurses provide holistic care to mothers and babies that includes patient education in areas of breast-feeding, diapering and bathing, umbilical cord care, and other safety areas in infant care. The mother/baby nurse also offers emotional support to mothers and their families, which is needed for a successful transition to parenthood. They must also be well versed in dealing with neonatal and maternal emergency situations.

EDUCATIONAL REQUIREMENTS

A registered nurse license is required; Bachelor of Science in Nursing is highly preferred; an experience in maternity or labor and delivery is highly desirable.

CORE COMPETENCIES/SKILLS NEEDED

- Knowledge of obstetrics, childbearing, and neonatal nursing
- Excellent teaching and communication skills
- Ability to work with members of health care team
- Strong computer and documentation skills
- Strong assessment and analytical skills

RELATED WEB SITE AND PROFESSIONAL ORGANIZATION

- Association of Women's Health, Obstetric and Neonatal Nurses (www.awhonn.org)

115 ■ MAGNETIC RESONANCE IMAGING NURSE

BASIC DESCRIPTION

A magnetic resonance imaging (MRI) nurse specifically works to provide nursing care to patients, and often their families, undergoing an MRI procedure. An MRI is an imaging procedure that is used to view an organ or a body part that uses magnetic energy instead of radiation. He/she could oversee staff in an MRI unit/suite, and works in a variety of patient care settings that can include inpatient services or ambulatory care services and deals with all types of patient populations from children to older adults.

EDUCATIONAL REQUIREMENTS

Registered nurse preparation and Basic Life Support certification are required; certification as radiology nurse is available.

CORE COMPETENCIES/SKILLS NEEDED

- Knowledge of care of patients specifically undergoing an MRI procedure
- Strong organization, managerial, and leadership skills
- Excellent communication and interpersonal skills
- Strong assessment and critical thinking skills
- Computer literacy

RELATED WEB SITES AND PROFESSIONAL ORGANIZATIONS

- American Radiological Nurses Association (http://www.rsna.org/)
- Association for Radiologic and Imaging Nursing (https://www.arinursing.org/)

116 ■ NEONATAL NURSE

BASIC DESCRIPTION
Neonatal nurses care for full or preterm babies specifically during the first 28 days of life. Neonatal nurses work with healthy newborns, those that need special care, such as preterm babies, or neonates that need constant monitoring and are critically ill.

EDUCATIONAL REQUIREMENTS
Registered nurse preparation and experience with pediatrics is highly preferred but not required. Pediatric Advanced Life Support and Neonatal Advanced Life Support certifications are required in most positions. The National Certification Corporation offers certification in several neonatal nursing concentrations, and the American Association of Critical Nurses offers certification in Neonatal Critical Care Nursing.

CORE COMPETENCIES/SKILLS NEEDED
- Knowledge of special and unique needs of the neonates and pediatric clients
- Excellent interpersonal and communication skills in working with families
- Excellent organization skills
- Good grasps of math to accurately administer medications
- Excellent assessment and critical thinking skills

RELATED WEB SITES AND PROFESSIONAL ORGANIZATIONS
- National Association of Neonatal Nurses (http://www.nann.org/)
- The Academy of Neonatal Nursing (http://www.academyonline.org/)
- Association of Women's Health, Obstetric and Neonatal Nurses (www.awhonn.org)
- National Certification Corporation (http://www.nccwebsite.org/Certification/default.aspx)
- American Association of Critical Care Nurses (www.aacn.org)

117 ■ NEONATAL NURSE PRACTITIONER

BASIC DESCRIPTION

Neonatal nurse practitioners are advanced practice nurses who specialize in providing care to acutely ill babies in the neonatal intensive care unit (NICU). These nurses have advanced skills in physical and psychosocial assessment of the newborn, and handle transport of acutely ill babies. The environments in which neonatal nurse practitioners work are very intense and dramatic, often with nonstop action.

EDUCATIONAL REQUIREMENTS

Registered nurse preparation and Master of Science in Nursing with advanced practice certification as a neonatal nurse practitioner are required. Programs are generally 2 years in length. These programs are affiliated with major medical centers that are equipped to care for premature babies. Previous experience in the NICU is usually a requirement for admission to a neonatal nurse practitioner program.

CORE COMPETENCIES/SKILLS NEEDED

- Technical competency involving use of complex and computerized equipment
- Skill in regulating ventilators
- Hemodynamic monitoring skills
- Experiences and expertise in assessing and managing acutely ill babies
- Skill in obtaining blood samples from central intravenous lines
- Interpersonal competency dealing with patients and their families in life-threatening situations
- Ability to work with interdisciplinary teams
- Ability to support parents' decisions even when you do not agree
- Comfort working with very small babies

RELATED WEB SITES AND PROFESSIONAL ORGANIZATIONS

- American Association of Nurse Practitioners (www.aanp.org)
- Nurse Practitioner Support Services (www.nurse.net)
- Pediatric Critical Care Medicine (www.pedsccm.wust1.edu)
- Association of Women's Health, Obstetric and Neonatal Nurses (www.awhonn.org/)
- National Association of Neonatal Nurses (www.nann.org/)
- American Nurses Association Credentialing Center (www.ana.org)

118 ■ NEPHROLOGY NURSE

BASIC DESCRIPTION

A nephrology nurse works with patients who have acute or chronic renal failure. The nurse works with patients in all stages of renal disease and administers treatment such as peritoneal dialysis and hemodialysis in a variety of settings. Examples of places of employment include hospitals, outpatient clinics, dialysis settings, and patients' homes.

EDUCATIONAL REQUIREMENTS

Registered nurse preparation is required. Although not a requirement for employment, a certification in dialysis nursing is helpful. On-the-job training is a large part of becoming adept at dialysis nursing. It takes approximately 6 weeks to train a nurse with experience and about 6 months before nurses are truly comfortable and able to troubleshoot problems effectively.

CORE COMPETENCIES/SKILLS NEEDED

- Ability to assess even very subtle changes in the condition of a dialysis/nephrology patient
- Ability to understand and operate equipment used for hemodialysis
- Excellent interpersonal and communication skills, especially when working with patients and their families as they deal with chronic renal disease and its impact
- Ability to teach patients about renal disease, treatment, and life-style changes
- Ability to deal with grief and loss that can be associated with renal disease
- Collaboration and teamwork

RELATED WEB SITE AND PROFESSIONAL ORGANIZATION

- American Nephrology Nurses' Association (www.annanurse.org)

119 ■ NEPHROLOGY NURSE PRACTITIONER

BASIC DESCRIPTION
A nephrology nurse practitioner provides primary care to patients with acute or chronic kidney/urologic disorders, those undergoing dialysis, and those who are candidates for or have undergone kidney transplants.

EDUCATIONAL REQUIREMENTS
Registered nurse preparation and Nurse Practitioner certification are required; certification is offered by the Nephrology Nursing Certification Commission.

CORE COMPETENCIES/SKILLS NEEDED
- Advanced knowledge in nephrology that includes pathophysiology and management of kidney/urologic conditions and their complications
- Excellent interpersonal, communication, and assessment skills
- Sensitivity to the needs of patients and their families as they deal with chronic renal disease and its impact
- Ability to teach patients about renal disease, treatment, and life-style changes
- Ability to deal with grief and loss that can be associated with renal disease
- Ability to work in a multidisciplinary team

RELATED WEB SITES AND PROFESSIONAL ORGANIZATIONS
- Nephrology Nursing Certification Commission (http://www.nncc-exam.org/cgi-bin/WebObjects/NNCCMain)
- American Nephrology Nurses Association (http://www.annanurse.org/cgi-bin/WebObjects/ANNANurse.woa)

120 ■ NEUROSCIENCE NURSE

BASIC DESCRIPTION

Neuroscience nurses take care of individuals who have experienced changes in function or alterations in consciousness and cognition communication, mobility, rest and sleep, sensations, and sexuality. A nurse working in the neuroscience field should enjoy technology and working with people, and have both physical and psychological stamina.

EDUCATIONAL REQUIREMENTS

Registered nurse preparation is required. Certification is available from the American Board of Neuroscience Nursing.

CORE COMPETENCIES/SKILLS NEEDED

- Skills in patient and family education, especially regarding the neurological condition
- Skill in using the nursing process to plan and implement care
- Knowledge of neuroscience nursing, including anatomy and physiology, illness manifestations, and medical treatments
- Ability to manage families and individuals who are grieving loss
- Technological skills

RELATED WEB SITES AND PROFESSIONAL ORGANIZATIONS

- American Association of Neuroscience Nurses (www.aann.org)
- American Association of Spinal Cord Injury Nurses (www.aascin.org)

121 ■ NURSE EXECUTIVE

BASIC DESCRIPTION
A nurse executive assumes a leadership role in a health care organization. She/he designs the institution's delivery of nursing care, plans and develops policies and procedures, assumes leadership in planning for the department's budget and fiscal needs, ensures adequate staffing, evaluates mid-level managers, and collaborates with other department heads.

EDUCATIONAL REQUIREMENTS
Registered nurse preparation and bachelor's degree, or higher, are required; certification is available from the American Nurses Credentialing Center.

CORE COMPETENCIES/SKILLS NEEDED
- Excellent leadership and management skills
- Strong communication and interpersonal skills
- Ability to work with members of other departments
- Knowledge related to budget and fiscal management
- Knowledge of leadership and management theories
- Knowledge and understanding of state and federal health care–related regulations
- Familiarity with Medicare, Medicaid, and third-party reimbursement
- Flexibility and ability to make quick decisions
- Objectivity, assertiveness, and excellent time management and organizational skills

RELATED WEB SITES AND PROFESSIONAL ORGANIZATIONS
- The American Organization of Nurse Executives (http://www.aone.org/)
- American Nurses Credentialing Center (www.nursecredentialingcenter.com)

122 ■ NURSE MANAGER

BASIC DESCRIPTION
A nurse manager responsibilities of a certain patient care unit or a practice setting. A nurse manager has administrative and clinical responsibilities and mediates between staff and upper-level management. The employer outlines the nurse manager's responsibilities.

EDUCATIONAL REQUIREMENTS
Registered nurse preparation and a master's preparation in nursing or management are highly preferred.

CORE COMPETENCIES/SKILLS NEEDED
- Excellent communication and interpersonal skills
- Advanced knowledge required based on area of specialization
- Knowledge of leadership and management principles
- Knowledge of the organization's policies and quality improvement process
- Knowledge of state and federal accreditation guidelines
- Knowledge of budgeting and other fiscal-related matters

RELATED WEB SITES AND PROFESSIONAL ORGANIZATIONS
- The Healthcare Performance Institute (http://www.healthcareperformanceinstitute.com/)
- The American Organization of Nurse Executives (http://www.aone.org/)

123 ■ NURSE MIDWIFE

BASIC DESCRIPTION
Certified nurse midwives are advanced practice nurses who specialize in providing care to healthy women during pregnancy, childbirth, and after birth. Midwives provide accessible, safe birth care especially in rural and inner city areas. They teach patients and their families about the birthing process and provide the mother in labor birthing information and individualized attention. They provide care in a variety of settings including hospitals, birthing centers, clinics, homes, and offices.

EDUCATIONAL REQUIREMENTS
Registered nurse preparation plus a baccalaureate degree (not necessarily in nursing) are required to become a nurse midwife. There are prerequisites that must be met but vary from one organization to another. The typical program averages 12 months, and a master's degree is the usual degree earned. The certification examination for nurse midwives is offered through the American College of Nurse-Midwives Certification Council.

CORE COMPETENCIES/SKILLS NEEDED
- Strong assessment skills specifically related to this specialty
- Good communication ability
- Excellent leadership and organizational skills
- Understanding of relevant technology
- Ability to collaborate with other members of the health care team
- Compassion and caring attitude
- Ability to deal with a variety of people

RELATED WEB SITES AND PROFESSIONAL ORGANIZATIONS
- American College of Nurse-Midwives (www.acnm.org or www.midwife.org)
- American Midwifery Certification Board (www.amcbmidwife.org)
- Association of Women's Health, Obstetric and Neonatal Nurses (www.awhonn.org)

124 ■ NURSE PSYCHOTHERAPIST

BASIC DESCRIPTION

Nurse psychotherapists work in a therapeutic relationship with their patients on either a one-to-one basis or in small therapy groups. Therapists form therapeutic alliances with their patients in order to help them to decrease their symptoms and to return to preillness level of function. Nurse psychotherapists work in a variety of settings including hospitals, clinics, and independent practice.

EDUCATIONAL REQUIREMENTS

Registered nurse preparation plus a master's degree and preparation as an advanced practice nurse are required. National certification by the American Nurses Credentialing Center in the specialty is required.

CORE COMPETENCIES/SKILLS NEEDED

- Advanced clinical skills in the area of psychiatric/mental health nursing
- Ability to practice independently in areas such as medication management and psychotherapy
- Ability to integrate research and theory into the practice of psychotherapy
- Ability to provide individual psychotherapy and psychiatric assessment
- Ability to integrate nursing science, computer science, and informatics in the provision of care
- Works collaboratively with other specialty groups

RELATED WEB SITES AND PROFESSIONAL ORGANIZATIONS

- American Psychiatric Nurses Association (www.acapn.org)
- Society for Education and Research in Psychiatric Mental Health Nursing (www.ispn-psych.org)

125 ■ NURSING SUPERVISOR

BASIC DESCRIPTION

The nursing supervisor oversees nursing and provides clinical leadership in a health care facility; s/he implements and interprets institutional policies and could also be involved in recruitment activities and preparing budgets.

EDUCATIONAL REQUIREMENTS

Registered nurse preparation is required; Bachelor of Science in Nursing is required for most positions; Basic Life Support certification, Advanced Cardiac Life Support certification, and at least 2 years clinical experience are required.

CORE COMPETENCIES/SKILLS NEEDED

- Strong clinical and interpersonal skills
- Assertiveness and excellent leadership and managerial skills
- Knowledge of budgeting and accounting and leadership theories
- Strong computer skills and documentation skills
- Knowledge of collective bargaining agreement contracts
- Ability to work independently and make quick decisions
- Ability to work with other members of the health care team

RELATED WEB SITE AND PROFESSIONAL ORGANIZATION

- The American Organization of Nurse Executives (http://www. aone.org/)

126 ■ NUTRITION SUPPORT NURSE

BASIC DESCRIPTION
Nutrition support nurses play a major role in the maintenance of patients' nutritional health. While most patients are able to eat or may just require some encouragement and assistance, some patients are unable to meet their nutritional needs via the oral route. The provision of nutrition support, which includes enteral feeding (via the gastrointestinal tract) and total parenteral nutrition (via the venous circulation), allows maintenance or repletion of the nutritional status for this group of patients. Nutrition support is provided by a multidisciplinary team comprising nurse clinicians, dieticians, gastroenterologists, surgeons, and pharmacists. The nurse clinician and team coordinate, provide, and advise patients on nutrition support. The team ensures that patients' nutritional needs are met by the safest, most economical, and most efficacious nutritional modality. Often the work includes assistance for children who require special nutritional intervention, including those with feeding disorders, growth failure, dietary intolerance, short bowel syndrome and congenital bowel disorders, and malabsorption. Nutrition support services can be provided to administer long-term intravenous nutrition or specialized tube feedings in selected cases.

EDUCATIONAL REQUIREMENTS
Registered nurse preparation is required. Certification is offered by the National Board of Nutrition Support Certification by the American Society for Parenteral and Enteral Nutrition.

CORE COMPETENCIES/SKILLS NEEDED
- Skill in developing guidelines and protocols on patient nutrition support
- Ability to manage the various acute and chronic nutritional access devices, both enteral as well as parenteral

- Skill in developing, implementing, and evaluating appropriate programs for staff training and patient teaching
- Interdisciplinary team skills
- Ability to work in a range of health care settings

RELATED WEB SITES AND PROFESSIONAL ORGANIZATIONS

- American Society for Parenteral and Enteral Nutrition (www.nutritioncare.org/)
- National Board of Nutrition Support Certification by the American Society for Parenteral and Enteral Nutrition (www.nutritioncertify.org)

127 ■ OCCUPATIONAL/INDUSTRIAL NURSE

BASIC DESCRIPTION
Occupational health nurses work in a variety of settings to keep workers healthy and to prevent work-related injuries. These nurses provide direct care services to employees on the job, host health promotion activities, and provide workers' compensation case management. This nurse is also often responsible for treatment of hazards in specific work environments. Practice settings include businesses, industries, government facilities, and shopping malls.

EDUCATIONAL REQUIREMENTS
Registered nurse preparation is required; Bachelor of Science in Nursing is often preferred, and graduate education may be required. Usually 2 years of medical/surgical experience is required. Certification in specialized occupational health nursing roles is available from the American Board for Occupational Health Nurses, Inc.

CORE COMPETENCIES/SKILLS NEEDED
- Knowledge of Occupational Safety and Health Administration (OSHA) regulations and workers' compensation laws
- Ability to maintain, protect, and preserve the health of employees in their work environment
- Ability to analyze and prioritize risk factors to achieve highest level of health among employees
- Ability to coordinate care
- Assist in meeting OSHA standards
- Ability to provide health education
- Ability to manage crises/emergencies
- Autonomy

- Innovative thinker
- Good communication skills
- Excellent health assessment skills
- Effective manager

RELATED WEB SITES AND PROFESSIONAL ORGANIZATIONS

- American Association of Occupational Health Nurses, Inc. (www.aaohn.org)
- American Board for Occupational Health Nurses, Inc. (www.abohn.org)

128 ■ OCCUPATIONAL HEALTH NURSE PRACTITIONER

BASIC DESCRIPTION

Occupational health nurse practitioners work with employees to ensure safe workplace conditions by conducting routine physical assessment, educating workers about hazard control, providing vaccinations, and counseling on health-promoting lifestyle. They make important recommendations to organizations that could lead to increased employee retention and job satisfaction.

EDUCATIONAL REQUIREMENTS

Registered nurse (RN) preparation, Nurse Practitioner certification, and Basic Life Support certification are required; clinical experience as an RN in ambulatory or acute care settings is required; certification is available from the American Board for Occupational Health Nurses.

CORE COMPETENCIES/SKILLS NEEDED

- Knowledge of workplace regulations such as those outlined by the Occupational Safety and Health Administration, Health Insurance Portability and Accountability Act, and the Family and Medical Leave Act
- Excellent interpersonal and communication skills
- Strong computer and documentation skills
- Strong organizational skills

RELATED WEB SITES AND PROFESSIONAL ORGANIZATIONS

- American Association of Occupational Health Nurses (https://www.aaohn.org/)
- American Board for Occupational Health Nurses (https://www.aaohn.org/)

129 ■ OFFICE NURSE

BASIC DESCRIPTION

Office nurses perform routine administrative and clinical tasks to keep the offices and clinics of family practice physicians, internal medicine, oncologists, cardiologists, surgeons, advanced practice nurses, and others running smoothly. The goal of the office nurse is to provide personalized and efficient service to the patients they serve. They often play an important role in uncovering problems or concerns of the patient and alerting the physician of these issues. They perform telephone triage and provide patient education about many routine topics. They care for the patients in offices, clinics, surgical centers, and emergency medical centers. Depending on the type of facility, the office nurse serves patients with a variety of needs—diagnostic, medication, monitoring, wound treatment, maintenance, preventive medicine, surgery, and education. One of the most important responsibilities of an office nurse is telephone triage, integrating appropriate attention to biological and psychosocial issues with high-quality medical care. Another vital role for office nurses is that of patient advocate. Duties vary from office to office, depending on location, size, and specialty. Administrative duties often include answering telephones, greeting patients, updating and filing patient medical records, filling out insurance forms, handling correspondence, scheduling appointments, arranging for hospital admission and laboratory services, and handling billing and bookkeeping.

EDUCATIONAL REQUIREMENTS

Registered nurse preparation is required; experience is often a major requirement, but there are classes available to enhance telephone triage skills.

CORE COMPETENCIES/SKILLS NEEDED
- Good communication skills
- Knowledge of disease processes and normal development

- Office management skills
- History taking and physical assessment skills
- Patient and family education
- Knowledge of medications
- Skill in routine nursing activities such as dressing changes, vital signs, and assessment

RELATED WEB SITE AND PROFESSIONAL ORGANIZATION

- The American Association of Office Nurses (www.aaon.org/)

130 ■ OMBUDSMAN

BASIC DESCRIPTION

An ombudsman is someone who investigates reported complaints, reports findings, and helps achieve equitable settlements. They handle complaints and concerns regarding the quality of life and the quality of care of vulnerable adults receiving long-term care services. Activities they perform include information and referral, problem solving, conflict resolution, mediation, and education. Because of the nature and diversity of the complaints and concerns, there is a need to work with many state and local organizations. The sources of the complaints are varied from the client themselves, to their families, provider staff, doctors, reps from state agencies, and hospital discharge planners. The complaints range from straightforward to multifaceted. For example, some need specialized equipment, and some have restraint concerns. Complaints may also include inadequate staffing, financial exploitation, alleged staff abuse, family conflicts, cold food, lost laundry, poor infection control, and decubitus ulcers. An ombudsman works with the department of health, the regulatory agency for all health care facilities in the long-term care continuum. They are often closely involved with the departments of elderly affairs, human services, and mental health and retardation, and hospitals, as they are providers and payers of care to the targeted population. They also work closely with the state's attorney general's office, attorneys, and the probate court system. As part of an organization, there is involvement in many committees, task forces, and councils, leading to legislative activities.

EDUCATIONAL REQUIREMENTS

Registered nurse preparation is required; nursing background and experience is of benefit because of many concerns regarding clinical issues. It is also beneficial to have nursing input due to the high acuity levels of people receiving long-term care services along with the dealings with the hospitals, the medical community, and the nursing industry at all levels. Families and clients also feel added reassurance that a nurse is involved.

CORE COMPETENCIES/SKILLS NEEDED
- Excellent listening and interpersonal skills
- Skill in documentation
- Flexibility
- Ability to work with individuals from a variety of backgrounds
- Management skills required for dealing with a large number of agencies and representatives

RELATED WEB SITES AND PROFESSIONAL ORGANIZATIONS
- The Ombudsman Association (www.ombuds-toa.org/)
- United States Ombudsman Association (www.usombudsman.org)

131 ■ ONCOLOGY NURSE

BASIC DESCRIPTION
An oncology nurse cares for patients with cancer in various stages of the disease. Most patients experience problems from both the disease and the treatment. Oncology nurses administer chemotherapy, manage symptoms and the effects of treatment, and care for the needs of their patients with empathy. They must also deal with the psychological ramifications that the diagnosis of cancer brings as well as with the issues related to death and dying. Oncology nurses may be employed in a variety of settings. They most often work in special oncology units within hospitals, but may work in outpatient areas, home care, and hospice care.

EDUCATIONAL REQUIREMENTS
Registered nurse preparation is required; a Bachelor of Science in Nursing or a higher degree in nursing may be required. Some agencies may require certification as an oncology nurse.

CORE COMPETENCIES/SKILLS NEEDED
- Ability to cope with human suffering, emergencies, and other stresses
- Maturity
- Excellent interpersonal and communication skills
- Strong teaching ability
- Able to adapt to new treatment regimens
- Knowledge of drugs used in chemotherapy is essential
- Strong knowledge background in disease processes and symptom management in particular forms of cancer

RELATED WEB SITES AND PROFESSIONAL ORGANIZATIONS
- Oncology Nursing Society (www.ons.org)
- Oncology Nursing Certification Corporation (www.oncc.org)
- Association of Pediatric Oncology Nurses (www.apon.org/)

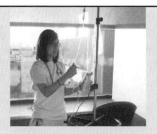

Profile:
JILL SAN JUAN
Oncology Nurse

1. What is your educational background in nursing (and other areas) and what formal credentials do you hold?

I graduated in 2009 with a Bachelors of Science in Nursing. I am a registered nurse in Ohio and Texas. As a nurse working on an oncology floor (more specifically, a leukemia unit), I am also certified in administering chemotherapy and vesicants.

2. How did you first become interested in the career that you are currently in?

In high school, community service hours were required for each year. I volunteered at a local hospital and was introduced to bedside interaction with patients. With oncology, I first became interested in the field during a summer externship of my junior year. I appreciated the technical and emotional aspects of the field. Oncology is fast paced and requires a high level of critical thinking. It is also an area where you build a special bond with your patients and families.

3. What are the most rewarding aspects of your career?

The most rewarding aspect of my oncology career is being by the patient and families from new diagnoses and throughout treatment. The continuity of care in oncology is unique because a typical hospital stay for a patient is a month (from being newly diagnosed and throughout whichever treatment they choose). Staff members on the floor really invest themselves in the patients, get to know them very well, and can become their sole support system. It is extremely

Continued

Profile: JILL SAN JUAN Continued

rewarding to see your patient come back and visit the staff on the unit just to tell you thank you for all that you do. This has happened many times!

4. What advice would you give to someone contemplating the same career path in nursing?

Nursing is an evolving career. Nursing is not limited to being in a hospital setting. A nurse can expand to teaching classes at nursing schools to working at a village in South America. Nursing is an extremely rewarding career for you and your patients. It is an area for personal growth. There are always opportunities to advance in your career if you are ready for a change.

132 ■ ONCOLOGY NURSE PRACTITIONER

BASIC DESCRIPTION
As primary care providers, oncology nurse practitioners (NPs) provide comprehensive care to patients who have a diagnosis of cancer, as well as to their families. In collaboration with health care team members, the oncology NP conducts a thorough physical assessment, writes prescriptions for medications, administers therapeutic measures, and evaluates care provided.

EDUCATIONAL REQUIREMENTS
Registered nurse preparation and NP certification are required; there are several certifications available for oncology NPs such as the Advanced Oncology Certified Nurse Practitioner and Advanced Oncology Certified Nurse Specialist by the Oncology Nursing Certification Corporation.

CORE COMPETENCIES/SKILLS NEEDED
- Excellent assessment, leadership, and critical thinking skills
- Ability to work with members of the health care team
- Excellent organization and fiscal skills

RELATED WEB SITES AND PROFESSIONAL ORGANIZATIONS
- Oncology Nursing Certification Corporation (http://www.oncc. org/TakeTest/Certifications/AOCNP)
- Oncology Nursing Society (http://www.ons.org/)

133 ■ OPHTHALMIC NURSE

BASIC DESCRIPTION
An ophthalmic nurse cares for patients with disorders and disease relating to the eyes. Ophthalmic nursing is full of opportunities for dedicated and highly skilled nurses who want to work with patients with ophthalmic diseases. Although it is a specialized field, it is also a career full of opportunities for nurses who want to use their general nursing knowledge and skills. Work settings include ophthalmologists' offices, hospitals, day surgery centers, research laboratories, and eye banks.

EDUCATIONAL REQUIREMENTS
Registered nurse preparation is required. The National Certifying Board for Ophthalmic Registered Nurses is an independently incorporated organization supported by the American Society of Ophthalmic Registered Nurses for the purpose of developing and implementing the certifying process for ophthalmic registered nurses. Candidates who meet the following criteria are eligible to take the certification examination for ophthalmic registered nurses: currently licensed as a registered nurse in the United States or having the equivalent hours (4,000) experience in ophthalmic registered nursing practice; completion and filing of an application for certification examination for ophthalmic registered nurses.

CORE COMPETENCIES/SKILLS NEEDED
- Ability to provide psychosocial support for patients and families
- Excellent communication skills
- Understanding of diseases of the eye and treatment protocols
- Ability to work in the operating room to assist with operative procedures

RELATED WEB SITE AND PROFESSIONAL ORGANIZATION
- American Society of Ophthalmic Registered Nurses (www.webeye.ophth.uiowa.edu/asorn/)
- National Certifying Board for Ophthalmic Registered Nurses (www.asorn.org)

134 ■ OR NURSE/PERIOPERATIVE NURSE

BASIC DESCRIPTION

A perioperative nurse or operating room (OR) nurse is a member of a surgical team that provides care for a patient before, during, and immediately after the patient has experienced a surgical intervention.

EDUCATIONAL REQUIREMENTS

Registered nurse preparation is required. Certification is available through the Association of Operating Room Nurses or from the Competency and Credentialing Institute.

CORE COMPETENCIES/SKILLS NEEDED

- Knowledge and skills needed to assist in preparing and operating the technological tools involved in new surgical techniques now available (e.g., lighter fiberoptic scopes/lenses and video monitors)
- Skill in providing comfort measures to the patient
- Skill in assisting the anesthetic caregivers
- Respect for cultural diversity, patients rights, privacy, and confidentiality
- Team skills for interactions with surgeons, surgical technologists, other nurses, anesthesiologists, nurse anesthetists, pathologists, radiologists, perfusionists, support assistant staff, and many other members of the health care team
- Skill in facilitating patient advocacy
- Excellent basic nursing skills in observation and assessment

RELATED WEB SITES AND PROFESSIONAL ORGANIZATIONS

- The Association of periOperative Registered Nurses (www.aorn.org)
- Competency and Credentialing Institute (www.cc-institute.org)

135 ■ ORGAN DONATION COUNSELOR

BASIC DESCRIPTION

An organ donation specialist/counselor is a nurse who works with families who have loved ones with irrevocable injuries on life support, and discusses the possibility of organ donation. There is a critical shortage of tissue and organ donation for transplants, and nurses can play a vital role in eliminating this shortage. Organ donation nurses are highly specialized and there are many related responsibilities. The education of nurses as designated requesters may have a considerable impact on the number of donors, because nurses are close to prospective donors and their families. Nurses provide a vital connection in the organ donation process.

EDUCATIONAL REQUIREMENTS

Registered nurse preparation is required. There are many programs that educate nurses to become donation requestors. The American Board of Transplant Coordinators offers two certifications to transplant coordinators after working in the field for a minimum of 1 year. Certification is available as either a Certified Procurement Transplant Coordinator or a Certified Clinical Transplant Coordinator.

CORE COMPETENCIES/SKILLS NEEDED

- Maturity
- Familiarity with types of donation and donation criteria
- Knowledge of the agency policy
- Knowledge of the types of transplantations
- Familiarity with different religious positions regarding tissue and organ donation
- Ability to deal with issues related to death and dying

RELATED WEB SITES AND PROFESSIONAL ORGANIZATIONS

- International Transplant Nurses Society (www.itns.org/)
- North American Transplant Coordinators' Organization (www.natco1.org/)

136 ■ ORTHOPEDIC NURSE

BASIC DESCRIPTION
Orthopedic nurses care for patients of all ages with actual and potential musculoskeletal injuries and conditions. An orthopedic nurse may provide assessments and educate patients about braces, prosthetics, and other orthopedic equipment. The nurse must be interested in the care of patients before and after surgery involving the musculoskeletal system such as total hip replacement, arthroscopy, total knee replacement, or spinal surgery. Orthopedic nursing is full of opportunities for dedicated and highly skilled nurses who want to work with patients with orthopedic conditions. Work settings include sports medicine clinics, sports franchises, hospitals, clinics, and day surgery centers.

EDUCATIONAL REQUIREMENTS
Registered nurse preparation is required. The Orthopaedic Nurses Certification Board provides a credentialing mechanism that validates proficiency in orthopedic nursing practice. Candidates who meet the following criteria are eligible to take the examination: currently licensed as a registered nurse, 2 years of professional nursing practice, and having a minimum of 1,000 hours of work experience in orthopedic nursing within the last 3 years.

CORE COMPETENCIES/SKILLS NEEDED
- Excellent communication skills
- Understanding of the laws of physics
- Interest in sports and physical activity

RELATED WEB SITES AND PROFESSIONAL ORGANIZATIONS
- National Association of Orthopedic Nurses (www.orthonurse.org)
- Orthopaedic Nurses Certification Board (www.oncb.org)

137 ■ PAIN MANAGEMENT NURSE

BASIC DESCRIPTION
The pain management nurse collaborates with an interdisciplinary team in the management of patients with acute and chronic pain. Pain management is a Joint Commission on Accreditation standard and is a critical need of many patients. Opportunities exist to work in acute care settings, outpatient clinics, rehabilitation centers, and home care.

EDUCATIONAL REQUIREMENTS
Registered nurse preparation is required. Certification in pain management is available from the American Nurses Credentialing Center and from the American Academy of Pain Management.

CORE COMPETENCIES/SKILLS NEEDED
- Empathy and understanding
- Understanding of the physiological and psychological aspects of pain
- Excellent communication skills
- Ability to work with interdisciplinary teams
- Interest in the complex issues regarding pain and the control of pain

RELATED WEB SITES AND PROFESSIONAL ORGANIZATIONS
- Pain Management and Nursing Role/Core Competency: A Guide for Nurses (www.dhmh.state.md.us/mbn/practice/pain_management.pdf)
- American Society of Pain Management Nurses (www.aspmn.org)
- American Nurses Credentialing Center (www.nursecredentialing. org)
- American Academy of Pain Management (www.aapainmanage.org)

138 ■ PAIN MANAGEMENT NURSE PRACTITIONER

BASIC DESCRIPTION
A pain management nurse practitioner provides a holistic approach in assessing, diagnosing, and managing acute and chronic pain across all age groups in variety of health care settings. The pain management nurse practitioner incorporates evidence-based approaches in implementing pharmacological and nonpharmacological interventions to alleviate pain and its associated symptoms.

EDUCATIONAL REQUIREMENTS
Registered nurse preparation, Nurse Practitioner certification, and Basic Life Support certification are required.

CORE COMPETENCIES/SKILLS NEEDED
- Sensitivity in dealing with patients and families
- Knowledge of palliative nursing and end-of-life care
- Excellent interpersonal and communication skills
- Excellent assessment and analytical skills and ability to work with the pain management team
- Excellent clinical and technical skills such as phlebotomy and medication administration

RELATED WEB SITES AND PROFESSIONAL ORGANIZATIONS
- American Society for Pain Management Nursing (http://www.aspmn.org/Organization/mission.htm)
- American Pain Society (http://www.ampainsoc.org/)

139 ■ PALLIATIVE CARE NURSE PRACTITIONER

BASIC DESCRIPTION
A palliative care nurse practitioner provides comprehensive care to patients and families living with a terminal illness. They could develop practice protocols for end-of-life care, educate other clinicians about palliative care, conduct research to expand knowledge about palliative care, and assume administrative roles in health care organizations.

EDUCATIONAL REQUIREMENTS
Registered nurse license and Nurse Practitioner certification are required; most positions require 1 year of acute care experience; certification is offered by the National Board for Certification of Hospice and Palliative Nurses.

CORE COMPETENCIES/SKILLS NEEDED
- Advanced knowledge and preparation in pain and symptom management and end-of-life care
- Sensitivity to the needs of terminally ill patients and their families
- Knowledge of hospice regulations and standards of care
- Excellent communication and assessment skills
- Strong computer and documentation skills
- Ability to work with an interdisciplinary team that includes physicians, social workers, dietitians, and unlicensed assistive personnel

RELATED WEB SITES AND PROFESSIONAL ORGANIZATIONS
- Hospice and Palliative Nurses Association (www.hpna.org)
- National Board for Certification of Hospice and Palliative Nurses (www.nbchpn.org)
- Center for Advance Palliative Care (www.capc.org)

140 ■ PARISH NURSE

BASIC DESCRIPTION

A parish nurse is a registered nurse who facilitates the holistic health of a congregation by focusing on spiritual, emotional, and physical dimensions of a person. Parish nurses act as liaison and facilitator among church, community, and hospital, and work with clergy in meeting the physical and spiritual needs of members of a particular congregation. Activities of parish nurses include community screenings (e.g., taking blood pressures, patient teaching, making home visits, and counseling and patient advocacy).

EDUCATIONAL REQUIREMENTS

Registered nurse preparation is required.

CORE COMPETENCIES/SKILLS NEEDED
- Interest in helping members of a congregation maintain optimum levels of health and independent living
- Excellent communication skills
- Caring and compassionate
- Strong religious affiliation
- Patient and family education
- Excellent assessment skills
- Advocacy skills

RELATED WEB SITES AND PROFESSIONAL ORGANIZATIONS
- Health Ministries USA (www.pcusa.org/health/usa/parishnursing/parishnursing.htm)
- International Parish Nurse Resource Center (http://ipnrc.parish-nurses.org/index.phtml)
- North Central Region Health Ministries Network: About Parish Nurses and Health Ministries; Frequently Asked Questions (www.healthministries.net/FAQs.htm)

141 ■ PATIENT EDUCATION COORDINATOR

BASIC DESCRIPTION

The patient education coordinator is responsible for educating patients about their disease, medications, and all aspects of care needed following hospitalization or a clinic visit. Patient education is intended to help patients and families cope with a crisis, gather information, learn self-care, and use attitudes and strategies to promote optimal health. Patients who are well informed about their own health actively make their own health care decisions, are more likely to have better health overall and enjoy a better quality of life, have fewer illness-related complications, tend to be more compliant with medication and treatment regimens, and are less likely to be a drain on diminishing health care resources. Opportunities are available to work in hospitals, clinics, schools, health care organizations, and home health agencies.

EDUCATIONAL REQUIREMENTS

Registered nurse preparation with Bachelor of Science in Nursing is required; a Master of Science in Nursing is preferred in most settings.

CORE COMPETENCIES/SKILLS NEEDED

- Ability to teach and inspire others
- Maturity and dependability
- Excellent communication skills
- Ability to work with interdisciplinary teams
- Interest in teaching patients, and knowledgeable about pathophysiology and health promotion
- Teaching patients to manage acute and chronic illness
- Postoperative teaching
- Planning health education programs
- Preparation of teaching materials
- Development of patient teaching plans in a form that is

readily understood by the patient and pertinent to their unique circumstances

RELATED WEB SITES AND PROFESSIONAL ORGANIZATIONS

- Health Care Education Association (www.hcea-info.org/)
- National Council on Patient Information and Education (www. talkaboutrx.org/)
- Association of Community Health Nursing Educators (www.uncc. edu/achne/)
- United States Department of Health and Human Services (www. hhs.gov/)

142 ■ PATIENT REVIEW INSTRUMENT NURSE ASSESSOR

BASIC DESCRIPTION
This specialized long-term care nurse role is to assess the appropriateness of long-term care placement of patients. Assessment areas include the patient's physical, cognitive, and medical conditions. In some states, the PRI is used to determine skilled care needs of long-term care residents.

EDUCATIONAL REQUIREMENTS
A registered nurse license is required.

CORE COMPETENCIES/SKILLS NEEDED
- Knowledge of long-term care state and federal regulatory standards
- Excellent organizational and assessment skills
- Ability to communicate with members of the health care team and patient's family or significant others
- Knowledge of the health care needs of older adults

RELATED WEB SITES AND PROFESSIONAL ORGANIZATIONS
- Island Peer Review Organization (www.ipro.org)
- New York State Department of Health (www.nyhealth.gov)

143 ■ PEACE CORPS VOLUNTEER

BASIC DESCRIPTION
Peace Corps volunteer nurses are assigned to specific jobs in third world countries. The history of the Peace Corps is the story of tens of thousands of people who have served as volunteers since 1961. Their individual experiences have comprised a legacy of service that has become part of American history. There is a 27-month commitment. These health volunteers work in both rural and urban settings where they raise awareness about the need for health education and infrastructures for healthy environments. They work on a variety of health activities in the community, from educating and training in the areas of maternal/child health, basic nutrition, sanitation, oral rehydration therapy, and sexually transmitted diseases/AIDS to organizing fund-raisers and community groups to obtain needed health care materials. Volunteers construct wells, tap springs, build latrines, improve potable water storage facilities, and train local leaders to maintain water and sanitation systems and continue health programs after the volunteer departs. They teach in classrooms and model methodologies for teachers in local schools and undertake knowledge, attitude, and practice surveys; assist clinics and/or ministerial planning offices in pinpointing health needs; devise educational projects to address prevailing health conditions; assist in the marketing of messages aimed at improving local health practices; and carry out epidemiological studies.

EDUCATIONAL REQUIREMENTS
Registered nurse preparation is required.

CORE COMPETENCIES/SKILLS NEEDED
- Flexibility
- Patience
- Maturity
- Curiosity

- Enthusiasm for helping people
- Dedication
- Compassion
- An understanding of different cultures
- Desire to make a difference in a developing country
- Excellent clinical skills

RELATED WEB SITE AND PROFESSIONAL ORGANIZATION

- Peace Corps (www.peacecorps.gov)

144 ■ PEDIATRIC CARDIAC NURSE ANESTHETIST

BASIC DESCRIPTION

A pediatric cardiac nurse anesthetist is part of the pediatric cardiac anesthesia team responsible for the care of children undergoing cardiac surgery and other cardiovascular procedures such as electrophysiologic studies. The pediatric cardiac nurse anesthetist is responsible for meeting the patient and the family before the operation to explain what to expect during and after the procedure.

EDUCATIONAL REQUIREMENTS

Registered nurse preparation and certification as Certified Registered Nurse Anesthetist are required; experience in acute or emergency care is mostly required; Basic Life Support, Pediatric Advanced Life Support, and Advanced Cardiac Life Support certifications are required; certification is offered by the National Board on Certification and Recertification of Nurse Anesthetists.

CORE COMPETENCIES/SKILLS NEEDED
- Ability to work with members of the team
- Excellent communication skills and sensitivity when addressing the needs and concerns of the family and the patient
- Excellent assessment skills and advance knowledge in cardiovascular, pulmonary, and hemodynamic physiology, management, and pharmacology
- Ability to work in a high-stress environment that requires quick decisions in cases of emergency and sudden change in patients' hemodynamic status
- Patient care requires light-to-moderate lifting

RELATED WEB SITES AND PROFESSIONAL ORGANIZATIONS

- American Association of Nurse Anesthetists (http://www.aana.com/)
- International Federation of Nurse Anesthetists (http://ifna-int.org/ifna/news.php)
- National Board on Certification and Recertification of Nurse Anesthetists (http://www.nbcrna.com/)

145 ■ PEDIATRIC NURSE

BASIC DESCRIPTION
A pediatric nurse is responsible for the nursing care of patients from infancy to late teens. They work in varied health care settings that range from ambulatory centers to acute care facilities. They may also work in specialized settings such as surgery, cardiology, rehabilitation, and oncology.

EDUCATIONAL REQUIREMENTS
Registered nurse license and Basic Life Support certification are required; certification is offered either by the Pediatric Nursing Certification Board or by the American Nurses Credentialing Center after passing an exam and completing practice hours. The American Association of Critical Care Nurses offers a certification in Pediatric Critical Care Nursing.

CORE COMPETENCIES/SKILLS NEEDED
- Flexibility in working with pediatric patients and their families
- Knowledge of unique needs of pediatric patients including growth and development and common disease conditions
- A thorough orientation is required for those who have no pediatric experience especially among new graduates

RELATED WEB SITES AND PROFESSIONAL ORGANIZATIONS
- Society of Pediatric Nurses (www.pednurses.org)
- Pediatric Nursing Board Certification Board (www.pncb.org)
- American Nurses Credentialing Center (www.nursecredentialing.org)
- American Association of Critical Care Nursing Certification Corporation (www.cetcorp.org)

146 ■ PEDIATRIC NURSE ANESTHETIST

BASIC DESCRIPTION

A pediatric nurse anesthetist cares for children during surgery or other medical or surgical procedures. They work in collaboration with anesthesiologists and could be employed in many settings such as the operating room and ambulatory care centers. During the delivery of anesthesia, they monitor the patient's level of consciousness, body functions, and responses to the procedure and intervene if there is a need. They work with the patient and families to make the hospital stay as pleasant as possible.

EDUCATIONAL REQUIREMENTS

Registered nurse preparation and certification as Certified Registered Nurse Anesthetist are required; experience as a registered nurse in pediatrics is mostly required for most positions; certification is offered by the National Board on Certification and Recertification of Nurse Anesthetists.

CORE COMPETENCIES/SKILLS NEEDED

■ Excellent communication skills
■ Excellent assessment and analytical skills
■ Advanced knowledge in pediatrics and sedation

RELATED WEB SITES AND PROFESSIONAL ORGANIZATIONS

■ American Association of Nurse Anesthetists (http://www.aana. com/)
■ International Federation of Nurse Anesthetists (http://ifna-int. org/ifna/news.php)
■ National Board on Certification and Recertification of Nurse Anesthetists (http://www.nbcrna.com/)

147 ■ PEDIATRIC NURSE PRACTITIONER

BASIC DESCRIPTION

Pediatric nurse practitioners are advanced practice nurses who provide management of care for acutely and/or chronically ill pediatric patients. Hospitalization is frightening for a child, so the pediatric nurse specialist must know how to alleviate or assist in alleviating fears of children and their families. Children of a young age are often unable to express their emotions; therefore, it is the responsibility of the pediatric nurse specialist to be alert to and aware of unexpressed needs. Work settings include acute care settings, subacute care settings, long-term care facilities, home care agencies, health maintenance organizations, ambulatory care settings, and schools.

EDUCATIONAL REQUIREMENTS

Bachelor of Science in Nursing, advanced practice licensure, Master of Science in Nursing in pediatrics or family health, and Pediatric Advanced Life Support certification are required. Continuing education for maintenance of licensure is also a requirement. Certification is available from the American Nurses Credentialing Center. A certification as a pediatric clinical nurse specialist is also available from the American Nurses Credentialing Center.

CORE COMPETENCIES/SKILLS NEEDED
- Special knowledge of growth and development
- Knowledge of pediatric illnesses and their treatment
- Ability to function independently
- Ability to work with children and their families
- Ability to set priorities and work independently
- Collaboration with other health care providers

RELATED WEB SITES AND PROFESSIONAL ORGANIZATIONS

- National Association of Pediatric Nurse Practitioners (www. napnap.org)
- Association of Pediatric Oncology Nurses (www.apon.org)
- The National Certification Board of Pediatric Nurse Practitioners and Nurses (www.pnpcert.org)
- Society of Pediatric Nurses (www.pedsnurses.org)
- American Nurses Credentialing Center (www.nursecredentialing. org)

148 ■ PEDIATRIC ONCOLOGY NURSE

BASIC DESCRIPTION
The pediatric oncology nurse—a highly specialized and sensitive role—delivers care to those pediatric patients who are receiving cancer treatment. Specific responsibilities include preparing patients for chemotherapy, administering palliative treatment, and collaborating with other members of the health care team.

EDUCATIONAL REQUIREMENTS
Registered nurse license and Basic Life Support certification are required; Pediatric Advanced Life Support certification is required for most positions; certification is offered by the Oncology Nursing Certification Corporation.

CORE COMPETENCIES/SKILLS NEEDED
- Knowledge of pediatric oncology
- Knowledge of safe handling of chemotherapeutic drugs
- Excellent communication, interpersonal, and assessment skills
- Flexibility and sensitivity of the unique needs of the pediatric oncology patients

RELATED WEB SITES AND PROFESSIONAL ORGANIZATIONS
- Association of Pediatric Oncology Nurses (www.apon.org)
- Oncology Nursing Certification Corporation (www.oncc.org)
- Oncology Nursing Society (www.ons.org)

149 ■ PERFORMANCE IMPROVEMENT DIRECTOR

BASIC DESCRIPTION
The director of performance improvement is responsible for the design, implementation, and evaluation of quality and performance improvement activities of a health care organization.

EDUCATIONAL REQUIREMENTS
Registered nurse preparation is required; master's degree is required in most positions; Certified Professional in Healthcare Quality certification is highly preferred.

CORE COMPETENCIES/SKILLS NEEDED
- Strong statistical skills
- Knowledge of federal and state health regulation, accreditation
- Knowledge of health policy, budget and fiscal-related matters, case management, risk management, and infection control
- Knowledge of grant writing activities to fund initiatives
- Strong written and verbal communication skills

RELATED WEB SITES AND PROFESSIONAL ORGANIZATIONS
- Healthcare Quality Certification Board (http://www.cphq.org/)
- National Committee on Quality Assurance (http://www.cphq.org/)
- National Organization of Competency Assurance (http://www.noca.org/)

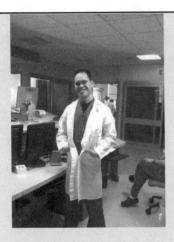

Profile:
JASON TAN
Performance Improvement
Coordinator

1. What is your educational background in nursing (and other areas) and what formal credentials do you hold?

I have a bachelor's degree in business administration and also a bachelor's degree in nursing, and a master's in business administration in quality management.

2. How did you first become interested in the career that you are currently in?

After finishing my first bachelors in business administration, I entered the corporate world. I was a stockbroker on Wall Street for a private firm. I then moved into banking. I left banking looking for something more meaningful. I wanted to be in a profession that would not only be gratifying but also something where I could grow as an individual professionally.

My mother, who has been an emergency room nurse for over 30 years, recommended that I consider a career in nursing. I originally was against it and had the stereotypical view that nursing was only for women. Through much research, volunteer work, and support of family and friends, I decided to go back to school to become a nurse.

Continued

Profile: JASON TAN Continued

3. What are the most rewarding aspects of your career?

It is rewarding to me to simply be able to help people day in and day out in their time of need. Every day brings a new challenge where I can leave my job knowing I was able to advance the health of a patient. The gratification from the patients is a reward in itself.

4. What advice would you give to someone contemplating the same career path in nursing?

Try to expose yourself to the multiple areas in nursing. Find an area that you can be passionate about and truly love. Learn as much as you can and pursue the direction you want to go in with the understanding that you will be helping someone in their time of need.

150 ■ PERIANESTHESIA NURSE

BASIC DESCRIPTION
Perianesthesia nursing provides intensive care to patients as they awake from anesthesia. The perianesthesia nurse prepares patients for the surgical experience, monitors and supports safe transition from anesthetized state to responsiveness, and readies patients for discharge from the perianesthesia care unit. They have opportunities to work in perianesthesia care units in inpatient and outpatient settings, including freestanding operative settings, hospitals, and clinics.

EDUCATIONAL REQUIREMENTS
Registered nurse preparation is required. Certification is available. There are two certification programs for qualified registered nurses: the CPAN program (Certified Post Anesthesia Nurse) and the CAPA program (Certified Ambulatory Perianesthesia Nurse).

CORE COMPETENCIES/SKILLS NEEDED
- Experience in medical–surgical and critical-care nursing
- Hands-on skills such as line placement, tube insertions, dressing changes, intravenous therapy, and positioning
- Flexibility
- Good assessment and decision-making skills
- Good management skills
- Technological ability
- Ability to teach
- Good interpersonal skills
- Must be able to respond to possible complications of anesthesia, including respiratory compromise, hypotension, emergence excitement, nausea and/or vomiting, and pain
- Must be flexible and have an ability to manage stress

RELATED WEB SITES AND PROFESSIONAL ORGANIZATIONS
- American Society of PeriAnesthesia Nurses (www.aspan.org)
- American Board of Perianesthesia Nursing Certification, Inc. (www.cpancapa.org)

151 ■ PERIOPERATIVE NURSE PRACTITIONER

BASIC DESCRIPTION
The primary responsibility of a perioperative nurse practitioner is to conduct a thorough physical assessment of patients scheduled for an operative procedure, screen for potential complications during and after surgery, order preoperative laboratory tests and interpret their results, and provide patient teaching and anticipatory guidance.

EDUCATIONAL REQUIREMENTS
Registered nurse preparation and Nurse Practitioner certification are required; Basic Life Support certification is required, and Advanced Cardiac Life Support certification is preferred in most positions; certification as adult nurse practitioner from the American Academy of Nurse Practitioners National Certification Program is available.

CORE COMPETENCIES/SKILLS NEEDED
- Excellent assessment and analytical skills
- Strong computer skills
- Ability to work in a fast-paced dynamic environment
- Ability to work in a team

RELATED WEB SITES AND PROFESSIONAL ORGANIZATIONS
- American Academy of Nurse Practitioners (http://www.aanp.org/AANPCMS2)
- Association of Perioperative Registered Nurses (www.aorn.org)

BASIC DESCRIPTION

A perinatal nurse cares for women, infants, and their families from the onset of pregnancy through the first month of the newborn's life (perinatal period). The perinatal nurse needs to convey to the provider the patient's physiological status (vital signs, contractions, physical examination findings) and the well-being of the fetus, as evidenced by fetal heart auscultation or monitoring, in clear language. Perinatal nurses have opportunities to work in hospitals including specialty hospitals, health departments, medical offices, health maintenance organizations, clinics, birthing centers, nurse midwife practices, and home health agencies.

EDUCATIONAL REQUIREMENTS

Registered nurse preparation is required. Certification in perinatal nursing is available.

CORE COMPETENCIES/SKILLS NEEDED

- Interpersonal skills
- Commitment
- Oral and written communication skills
- Ability to monitor the pregnancy
- Ability to assess the progression of labor and maintain a sense of calm and comfort during labor
- Ability to monitor the status of mother and baby
- Knowledge of family support
- Skill in fostering the new mother–infant relationship and teaching parenting skills

■ Ability to assess and support the mother in her recovery from childbirth as well as evaluate the newborn's early adjustment to life

RELATED WEB SITES AND PROFESSIONAL ORGANIZATIONS

■ Association of Women's Health, Obstetric and Neonatal Nurses (www.awhonn.org/)
■ National Association of Neonatal Nurses (www.nann.org/)
■ American Nurses Credentialing Center (www.nursingworld.org/ancc/)

153 ■ PHARMACEUTICAL REPRESENTATIVE

BASIC DESCRIPTION
The pharmaceutical representative is a registered nurse involved in promoting and selling products from pharmaceutical companies. Practice settings include pharmaceutical companies and telemarketing companies.

EDUCATIONAL REQUIREMENTS
Registered nurse preparation is required; some companies prefer Bachelor of Science in Nursing.

CORE COMPETENCIES/SKILLS NEEDED
- Knowledge of product being promoted
- Ability to manage time effectively
- Good organizational skills
- Marketing skills
- Professional demeanor
- Outgoing personality
- Good communication skills
- Self-motivated
- Ability to be flexible and travel

RELATED WEB SITES AND PROFESSIONAL ORGANIZATIONS
- Industry managers and recruiters provide credible advice on the Who, What, When, Where, Why, and How of breaking into pharmaceutical sales (www.pharmaceutical-sales-info.com/) (there is a $15 fee to register on this Web site)
- Pharmaceutical Representative Online (www.pharmrep.com/)

154 ■ PHARMACEUTICAL RESEARCH NURSE

BASIC DESCRIPTION
The pharmaceutical research nurse is involved in clinical trials that involve the use of pharmacological agents and could be tasked with overseeing the implementation of the research protocol that includes drug handling and dosing in consultation with the pharmacist and clinical researcher.

EDUCATIONAL REQUIREMENTS
Registered nurse preparation is required; Bachelor of Science in Nursing is required in most positions.

CORE COMPETENCIES/SKILLS NEEDED
- Strong phlebotomy skills
- Strong computer and documentation skills
- Excellent interpersonal and communication skills
- Knowledge of research process and Institutional Review Board protocol

RELATED WEB SITE AND PROFESSIONAL ORGANIZATION
- Pharmaceutical Research and Manufacturers of America (http://www.phrma.org/)

155 ■ PLASTIC AND RECONSTRUCTIVE SURGERY NURSE

BASIC DESCRIPTION

Plastic and reconstructive surgical nurses care for patients undergoing cosmetic surgery to correct esthetic problems (e.g., face lift, breast augmentation), or to reconstruct some part of the body from disease, accident, or malformations (e.g., skin lesions and tumors, congenital deformities, facial fractures, burns, ulcers, varicose veins, reconstruction after cancer surgery). There is often a great deal of patient happiness and appreciation following the surgery. Opportunities exist to work in hospitals, ambulatory surgery centers, and office practices.

EDUCATIONAL REQUIREMENTS

Registered nurse preparation is required. Certification is available as a Certified Plastic Surgical Nurse through the Plastic Surgical Nursing Certification Board, Inc.

CORE COMPETENCIES/SKILLS NEEDED
- Skills in patient care
- Specialized teaching about the patient's particular operative procedure
- Perioperative and postoperative care
- Excellent communication skills
- Consideration of clients' needs

RELATED WEB SITES AND PROFESSIONAL ORGANIZATIONS
- The American Society of Plastic and Reconstructive Surgical Nurses (www.karpinskimd.com/ASPRSN.html)
- American Society of Plastic Surgical Nurses (www.aspsn.org/)

210

156 ■ POISON INFORMATION NURSE

BASIC DESCRIPTION
Working with poison control centers, the poison information nurse provides education to individuals, organizations, and businesses regarding poison prevention and management.

EDUCATIONAL REQUIREMENTS
Registered nurse preparation is required; Basic Life Support certification is required in most positions.

CORE COMPETENCIES/SKILLS NEEDED
- Advanced knowledge of the effects of different types of poison on the body
- Ability to work in a dynamic and high-stress environment especially for those who are working in emergency departments
- Ability to provide sensitive and empathic care to patients, especially if cause is self-inflicted
- Excellent communication and documentation skills

RELATED WEB SITES AND PROFESSIONAL ORGANIZATIONS
- American Association of Poison Control Centers (http://www.aapcc.org/dnn/default.aspx)
- Agency for Toxic Substances and Disease Registry (http://www.atsdr.cdc.gov/)
- American Academy of Clinical Toxicology (http://www.clintox.org/index.cfm)

157 ■ PRIVATE DUTY NURSE

BASIC DESCRIPTION

Private duty nurses provide total individual patient care in the home or hospital environment with payment coming from a private source or insurance. Private duty nurses can work through an agency or independently.

EDUCATIONAL REQUIREMENTS

Registered nurse preparation is required.

CORE COMPETENCIES/SKILLS NEEDED

- Solid foundation in nursing skills
- Ability to assist patients with personal hygiene, activities of daily living, medication management, dressing changes, and intravenous therapy
- Ability to conduct complete assessments and monitoring when necessary
- Ability to provide emotional support
- Problem-solving skills

RELATED WEB SITES AND PROFESSIONAL ORGANIZATIONS

- No Web sites available.

158 ■ PSYCHIATRIC NURSE

BASIC DESCRIPTION

Psychiatric nursing is centered around meeting the health needs of patients, with a particular focus on mental health. Psychiatric nurses may work with patients in an inpatient hospital setting, or a range of outpatient and community-based health care settings. A psychiatric nurse uses therapeutic communication to help patients of all ages better understand themselves and make behavior changes. Patients who are seen by psychiatric nurses may have a variety of illnesses, such as psychoses, personality and mood disorders, substance abuse disorders, and depression, just to name a few. Psychiatric nurses may work with child, adolescent, or adult patients. Psychiatric nursing involves understanding not only the mental but also the biological aspects of human thought processes and behaviors. Pharmacology also plays a role in psychiatric nursing, because there are many different medications used to treat mental illness and nurses must understand the physiological effects of these medications. Psychiatric nurses may be prepared as advanced practice nurses and as psychotherapists.

EDUCATIONAL REQUIREMENTS

Registered nurse preparation is required. Past work experience in any setting where there was a focus on therapeutic communication is extremely important. A solid medical–surgical background with strong assessment experience is important in order to understand and recognize the physiological effects of psychiatric treatment. Certification is available as a psychiatric/mental health nurse, clinical specialist, or nurse practitioner through the American Nurses Credentialing Center; psychiatric nurses may be licensed as individual, family, or group therapists.

CORE COMPETENCIES/SKILLS NEEDED

- Excellent communication skills, because therapeutic communication is used in every encounter with patients

- Strong critical thinking skills
- Ability to work with child, adolescent, adult, and elderly patients
- Observation skills to recognize and understand a patient's nonverbal communication
- Excellent crisis management skills in order to handle potentially dangerous situations and protect themselves and their patients from harm
- Ability to deal with patients who may be uncooperative or even dangerous at times
- Ability to treat patients with a holistic, nonjudgmental attitude
- Values for mental health as an important aspect of the health care system
- Patient advocacy skills

RELATED WEB SITES AND PROFESSIONAL ORGANIZATIONS

- American Psychiatric Nurses Association (www.apna.org)
- Alliance for Psychosocial Nursing (www.psychnurse.org/)
- American Nurses Credentialing Center (www.nursingworld.org/ancc/index.htm)
- Association of Child and Adolescent Psychiatric Nurses (www.ispn-psych.org/html/acapn.html)

159 ■ PUBLIC AND COMMUNITY HEALTH NURSE

BASIC DESCRIPTION
Public health nurses and community health nurses provide individual and population-focused community-oriented care. Community nurses participate in assessing the population in order to determine needed health services with the goal to improve the overall health of the community through disease prevention, health promotion, and wellness/health education. The public health nurse's goal in general is to promote and protect the health of populations using social and public health, public health sciences, and knowledge from nursing. They may also be involved in community health fairs, educational events, and establishing relationships with community organizations. They often assume responsibility for personnel, resources, and patient care in public health and will develop, implement, and evaluate educational programs and activities designed to meet these needs. They may also be involved in one-on-one education, making follow-up phone calls, and conducting home visits, with appropriate documentation of these services. This person may also establish and control the budget and support standards of nursing in the public health practice.

EDUCATIONAL REQUIREMENTS
Registered nurse preparation is required. Certification as a community health nurse and as a clinical specialist in community health nursing is available through the American Nurses Credentialing Center.

CORE COMPETENCIES/SKILLS NEEDED
- Knowledge of public health and epidemiology
- Collaborative abilities and team skills
- Assertiveness and self-reliance
- Interpersonal skills
- Analytical skills

- Policy development skills
- Cultural competency
- Management skills
- Must enjoy team effort and providing service in the community

RELATED WEB SITES AND PROFESSIONAL ORGANIZATIONS

- American Public Health Association (www.apha.org)
- American Nurses Credentialing Center (www.nursecredential-ing.org)

160 ■ PUBLIC POLICY ADVISER

BASIC DESCRIPTION
In this role as a public policy adviser, the nurse provides organizations advice related to health care and policy to achieve goals at the local, regional, or national level.

EDUCATIONAL REQUIREMENTS
Registered nurse preparation and at least a master's degree in nursing, health-related field, or health policy.

CORE COMPETENCIES/SKILLS NEEDED
- Knowledge of health policy and legislative process
- Excellent interpersonal and communication skills
- Assertiveness and strong computer skills
- Flexibility with time and ability to travel
- Involvement with various nursing and health care organizations

RELATED WEB SITES AND PROFESSIONAL ORGANIZATIONS
- National League for Nursing (www.nln.org)
- American Nurses Association (www.ana.org)

161 ■ PULMONARY/RESPIRATORY NURSE

BASIC DESCRIPTION
A pulmonary and respiratory nurse promotes pulmonary health for individuals, families, and communities, and cares for persons with pulmonary dysfunction throughout the patient's life span. Respiratory nursing may be preventive, acute, critical, or rehabilitative. There are opportunities to work in hospitals, extended care centers, private companies, health departments, office practices, and clinics.

EDUCATIONAL REQUIREMENTS
Registered nurse preparation is required.

CORE COMPETENCIES/SKILLS NEEDED
- Knowledge of respiratory diseases such as asthma, chronic obstructive pulmonary disease, tuberculosis, cystic fibrosis, and respiratory failure
- Excellent patient and family relationships and teaching abilities
- Team skills to work with other members of the health care team
- Ability to deal with issues of grief and loss
- Strong assessment skills
- Knowledge of oxygen therapies, assisted ventilation, and suctioning
- Patience for patient nonadherence to regimen and tobacco abuse
- Ability to discuss smoking cessation techniques, ability to administer and teach pharmacological interventions

RELATED WEB SITES AND PROFESSIONAL ORGANIZATIONS
- Respiratory Nursing Society (www.respiratorynursingsociety.org)
- American Association of Cardiovascular and Pulmonary Rehabilitation (www.aacvpr.org)

162 ■ QUALITY ASSURANCE NURSE

BASIC DESCRIPTION
Nurses in quality assurance (QA) promote quality and cost-effective outcomes for an organization by interpreting and applying the policies and procedure guidelines. They must identify and coordinate the needs of the patients with needs of the provider and orchestrate patient care among multiple caregivers through the continuum from preadmission through discharge based on age and cultural and individual patient needs. These nurses support and act as liaisons with the payers, providers, and patients and serve as the primary patient information resource for payers. QA nurses collaborate with physicians and treatment teams to develop patient-care guidelines and serve on quality-improvement teams. There are QA opportunities to work in the private sector, hospitals, and government facilities.

EDUCATIONAL REQUIREMENTS
Registered nurse preparation is required; Bachelor of Science in Nursing is preferred. Certification from Healthcare Quality Certification Board is available.

CORE COMPETENCIES/SKILLS NEEDED
- Training or experience in utilization review, discharge planning, and case management
- Strong interpersonal and communication skills
- Acute care skills
- Ability to identify problems such as underutilization or overutilization of services
- Self-directed with positive attitude
- Ability to promote and maintain quality care through analysis

RELATED WEB SITES AND PROFESSIONAL ORGANIZATIONS
- Agency for Healthcare Research Quality (www.ahrq.gov)
- Joint Commission for Accreditation of Health Care Organizations (www.jcaho.org)
- Healthcare Quality Certification Board (www.cphq.org)

163 ■ RADIOLOGY NURSE

BASIC DESCRIPTION
Radiology nurses work primarily in the hospital setting, assisting, performing, and teaching in the role of radiological imaging. Contemporary radiology departments are equipped with state-of-the-art imaging capacities, and radiology nurses assist in the care of patients undergoing invasive procedures.

EDUCATIONAL REQUIREMENTS
Registered nurse preparation is required. Certification is available from the Radiologic Nursing Certification Board, Inc.

CORE COMPETENCIES/SKILLS NEEDED
- Strong anatomy and physiology theory base and education in disease processes of human body
- Technical proficiency and knowledge of procedures to be performed
- Good teaching skills to prepare and help clients reach best outcome from a test/procedure
- Good knowledge of body mechanics for optimal positioning of patient for procedure
- Ability to identify and interpret life-threatening arrhythmias
- Skill in reviewing patient's clinical history for potential indicators that might contraindicate the procedure
- Skills in advocating for patient safety

RELATED WEB SITES AND PROFESSIONAL ORGANIZATIONS
- Radiological Society of North American, Inc. (www.rsna.org)
- Radiologic Nursing Certification Board (www.ama.net)

164 ■ RAPID RESPONSE NURSE

BASIC DESCRIPTION

Rapid response nurses are part of an expert clinical team in the acute care area, whose main goal is to prevent deaths and arrest hemodynamic decline in patients outside of intensive care units. They are experts in assessment and have clinical skills in implementing early interventions to prevent cardiopulmonary arrest.

EDUCATIONAL REQUIREMENTS

Registered nurse preparation, Basic Life Support certification, and Advanced Cardiac Life Support certifications are required.

CORE COMPETENCIES/SKILLS NEEDED

- Excellent assessment and critical thinking skills
- Excellent clinical skills such as initiating intravenous access, defibrillation, and suctioning
- Ability to work in a highly dynamic environment and to quickly respond to urgent calls anywhere in the acute care facility
- Excellent communication skills while working with other members of the rapid response team

RELATED WEB SITE AND PROFESSIONAL ORGANIZATION

- Institute for Healthcare Improvement (http://www.ihi.org/IHI/Topics/CriticalCare/IntensiveCare/Tools/RapidResponseTeamEducationChecklist(IHITool).htm)

165 ■ RECOVERY ROOM NURSE

BASIC DESCRIPTION
As a highly skilled clinician, the recovery room nurse is responsible for monitoring immediate postoperative patients across age groups and works in varied health care settings such as acute care facilities and ambulatory care settings. The recovery room nurse is also responsible for ensuring that acute complications arising from surgery are prevented by intervening if acute life-threatening complications occur.

EDUCATIONAL REQUIREMENTS
A registered nurse license is required; Basic Life Support and Advanced Cardiac Life Support certifications are required; certification is available from the American Board of Perianesthesia Nursing Certification.

CORE COMPETENCIES/SKILLS NEEDED
- Excellent communication and assessment skills
- Knowledge of cardiovascular and respiratory physiology and pathophysiology, and critical care concepts
- Ability to make quick decisions regarding patient's clinical condition and make urgent referrals to physicians
- Ability to work under pressure
- Knowledge of telemetry and ventilator management

RELATED WEB SITES AND PROFESSIONAL ORGANIZATIONS
- American Board of Perianesthesia Nursing Certification (www.cpancapa.org)
- American Society of Perianesthesia Nurses (www.aspan.org)
- The Pre-Operative Association (www.pre-op.org)

166 ■ RECRUITER

BASIC DESCRIPTION
Nurse recruiters develop and implement short- and long-term recruitment plans and strategies to meet nurse staffing needs. They also create, coordinate, and maintain a wide range of cost-effective recruitment strategies to generate applicant pools and hires. Work settings include hospitals, nursing homes, schools of nursing, and travel health care companies.

EDUCATIONAL REQUIREMENTS
Registered nurse preparation is required.

CORE COMPETENCIES/SKILLS NEEDED
- Excellent interpersonal skills
- Ability to screen and interview prospective job applicants
- Ability to develop relationships with the various nursing programs/schools in the area to promote nursing career opportunities and market
- Ability to contact, interview, and place nurses in jobs at a health care facility
- Self-directed and self-motivated
- Team skills
- Marketing skills
- Excellent phone voice, positive and enthusiastic
- Organizational skills
- Focus with attention to detail

RELATED WEB SITES AND PROFESSIONAL ORGANIZATIONS
- National Association for Health Care Recruitment (www.nahcr.com/)
- Nurse Recruiter for Nurses by Nurses (www.nurse-recruiter.com)

167 ■ REHABILITATION NURSE

BASIC DESCRIPTION
Rehabilitation nursing is a specialty practice area that involves care of individuals with altered functional ability and altered lifestyle. Rehabilitation nurses begin to work with injured or ill individuals and their families soon after a disabling injury or chronic illness strikes, and they continue to provide support after these individuals go home or return to work or school. The goal of rehabilitation nursing is to assist individuals with disabilities and chronic illness in the restoration, maintenance, and promotion of optimal health. Rehabilitation nursing practice occurs in many settings and involves a variety of roles. Most opportunities exist in hospitals (including specialty hospitals), long-term care facilities, and freestanding facilities.

EDUCATIONAL REQUIREMENTS
Registered nurse preparation is required. A registered nurse with at least 2 years of practice in rehabilitation nursing can earn distinction as a Certified Rehabilitation Registered Nurse (CRRN) by successfully completing an examination that validates expertise. Likewise, a registered nurse with a CRRN and a master's degree or doctorate in nursing can earn certification as a CRRN-Advanced.

CORE COMPETENCIES/SKILLS NEEDED
- Long-term patient and colleague relationships
- Ability to work with clients from infancy to elderly
- Teamwork and collaboration
- Patient and family education
- Innovative thinking
- Autonomy and independence
- Skilled at treating alterations in functional ability and lifestyle resulting from injury, disability, and chronic illness
- Skill in providing comfort, therapy, and education

- Skill to promote health-conducive adjustments, support adaptive capabilities, and promote achievable independence
- Skill in promoting holistic, comprehensive, and compassionate end-of-life care, including promotion of comfort and relief of pain
- Excellent functional assessment skills
- Skill in team management as they act as multisystem integrators and team leaders, working with physicians, therapists, and others to solve problems and promote patients' maximal independence
- Ability to work with others to adapt ongoing care to the resources available distinguishes the practice of rehabilitation nursing
- Goal oriented and focused on helping patients return to optimal functionality
- Ability to provide holistic care to meet patients' medical, vocational, educational, environmental, and spiritual needs
- Ability to function not only as caregivers but also as coordinators, collaborators, counselors, and case managers

RELATED WEB SITE AND PROFESSIONAL ORGANIZATION

- Association of Rehabilitation Nurses (www.rehabnurse.org/)

168 ■ REPRODUCTIVE NURSE

BASIC DESCRIPTION

A reproductive nurse provides education and counseling to individuals and their family about fertility concerns and other reproduction-related concerns that include menopause, impotence, and other forms of sexual dysfunctions.

EDUCATIONAL REQUIREMENTS

Registered nurse preparation is required.

CORE COMPETENCIES/SKILLS NEEDED
- Sensitivity to patients and their families
- Excellent verbal and written communication skills
- Advance knowledge of the reproductive system physiology, pathophysiology, and disease management
- Strong computer skills and knowledge of electronic health record documentation

RELATED WEB SITES AND PROFESSIONAL ORGANIZATIONS
- Association of Reproductive Health Professionals (http://www.arhp.org/)
- North American Menopause Society (http://www.menopause.org/)
- American Society for Reproductive Medicine (http://www.asrm.org/)

169 ■ RESEARCH COORDINATOR

BASIC DESCRIPTION
A research coordinator performs a role that includes coordination and management and conducts clinical research under the supervision of a designated investigator. The research coordinator position may be undertaken with a wide range of scientific investigations (e.g., basic research, clinical research, and epidemiological research) under the direction of scientists from many health disciplines.

EDUCATIONAL REQUIREMENTS
Registered nurse preparation and licensure are required; undergraduate and graduate preparation and a background in participation in research are desirable.

CORE COMPETENCIES/SKILLS NEEDED
- Knowledge of the research process
- Knowledge of the ethical requirements for conducting research and the knowledge of the human subjects research requirements
- Organizational skills
- Writing and reporting skills, including proposal development skills to assist the investigator in preparing proposals and reports
- Ability to work under pressure to accomplish research goals
- Knowledge of potential funding agency requirements
- Skill at managing teams including data collectors, research assistants, and project investigators

RELATED WEB SITES AND PROFESSIONAL ORGANIZATIONS
- National Institutes of Health, Understanding Clinical Trials (http://clinicaltrials.gov/ct2/info/understand)
- Clinical Research Careers (http://sciencecareers.sciencemag.org/career_magazine/previous_issues/articles/2002_04_05/noDOI.15495717378751859676)

170 ■ RESEARCHER

BASIC DESCRIPTION
A nurse researcher conducts studies related to individual, family, and community health; symptoms of illness; and nursing interventions to promote health and decrease incidence or symptoms of illness and conducts research related to nursing and health care delivery including workforce planning. The research may involve a large project funded through the National Institutes of Health or a small project supported by funds from the researcher's institution. Research requires an attention to detail; thus, the work is methodical and sometimes tedious. Researchers may work alone or in teams with other nurse researchers or clinicians; often the research undertaken by nurse scientists is multidisciplinary in nature, thus requiring the researchers to engage in team building and team functioning. Researchers often work under great pressure to meet deadlines for funding agencies or publication deadlines.

EDUCATIONAL REQUIREMENTS
PhD degree in nursing or related discipline is required.

CORE COMPETENCIES/SKILLS NEEDED
- Research methods knowledge and skills
- Knowledge of statistical methods and analyses
- Grant writing skills
- Analytical and organizational skills
- Writing skills
- Team building skills are often required

RELATED WEB SITES AND PROFESSIONAL ORGANIZATIONS
- National Institute of Nursing Research; a branch of the US Health and Human Services National Institutes of Health (www.nih.gov/ninr/)
- Sigma Theta Tau International (www.nursingsociety.com)

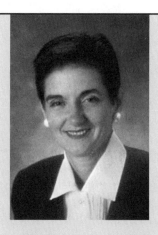

Profile:
MARY KERR
Nurse Researcher

1. What is your educational background in nursing (and other areas) and what formal credentials do you hold?

I have a diploma in nursing, a Bachelors of Science in Nursing (BSN), a Masters of Nursing Education, and a PhD in nursing.

2. How did you first become interested in the career that you are currently in?

I became interested in nursing in high school and was a member of the Future Nurses of America club. I became interested in research when I conducted a research project as part of my BSN—I counted microbes on gloves used in the operating room. I was intrigued by the idea of using data to examine and improve the outcomes of clinical care.

3. What are the most rewarding aspects of your career?

Each position that I held offered different rewards. Conducting research within an interdisciplinary, clinical environment was extremely challenging and intellectually stimulating. I also enjoyed teaching in an academic environment, helping students learn how to solve clinical problems by using data. Moving from academia to government was a fascinating change—now, as deputy director of the National Institute of Nursing Research (NINR), I get to see the benefits of nursing science applied to the health of the public on a national scale, which is deeply rewarding and enlightening. Throughout my career as a scientist, I have devoted myself to the training and mentoring of the next

Continued

Profile: MARY KERR Continued

generation of investigators. It has been most gratifying to work for a public institution that shares this goal and devotes a significant percentage of its resources toward developing new investigators.

4. What advice would you give to someone contemplating the same career path in nursing?

First, I would strongly recommend that, as freshmen, undergraduate nursing students participate in a research project headed by a nurse scientist. Whether they volunteer or are hired as student workers, the experience will help them determine if they might want to pursue a career as a nurse scientist. If they are interested in that path, the second step is applying to a PhD program in nursing research before they graduate. Next, rather than working full time and going to school part time, like the majority of nurses who seek advanced degrees, I would advise them to attend school full time and work as a nurse part time. This way everything they learn while pursuing their advanced degree will be integrated into their clinical practice.

To those who are already practicing nurses, I would encourage them to consider research, even if it means returning to school. Nursing science is coming into its own and, given the looming nurse faculty shortages, the field is wide open. Nurses, with their training in clinical observation and evaluation of patients, already have the basic skills that are critical for a research career; it is a natural next step to improve outcomes and help patients via research. Despite what many believe, pursuing a research career does not necessarily mean leaving patients behind. On the contrary, developing research projects with real-world benefits often requires regular interaction with patients. I encourage anyone who is interested in learning more about this field to visit the NINR Web site, which offers a condensed introductory nursing research course.

171 ■ RESPIRATORY NURSE PRACTITIONER

BASIC DESCRIPTION

Respiratory nurse practitioners deal with patients across age groups who have acute or chronic pulmonary disorders such as asthma, chronic obstructive pulmonary disorders, and cystic fibrosis; they work in various health care practice settings. Aside from providing primary care, they also educate patients with regard to prevention of future attacks and complications and participate in health promotion and maintenance activities.

EDUCATIONAL REQUIREMENTS

Registered nurse preparation and Nurse Practitioner certification are required; Basic Life Support and Advanced Cardiac Life Support certifications are required for most positions.

CORE COMPETENCIES/SKILLS NEEDED

- Knowledge of respiratory system's anatomy, physiology, and pathophysiology and their common treatments
- Excellent assessment and communication skills
- Knowledge of educational principles and experience in public speaking are highly desirable

RELATED WEB SITES AND PROFESSIONAL ORGANIZATIONS

- Respiratory Nursing Society (http://www.respiratorynursingsociety. org/index.html)
- American Association of Cardiovascular and Pulmonary Rehabilitation (www.aacvpr.org)

172 ■ RHEUMATOLOGY NURSE

BASIC DESCRIPTION
Rheumatology nurses provide care for patients suffering from diseases, such as arthritis, fibromyalgia, and myositis, that affect muscles, bones, and joints. Their goals are to provide interventions to relieve pain and prevent complications and to educate patients about health-promoting behaviors to decrease pain symptoms and prevent complications. They work in various health care settings such as acute care facilities, ambulatory centers, and specialized rheumatology clinics.

EDUCATIONAL REQUIREMENTS
Registered nurse certification and Basic Life Support certification are required.

CORE COMPETENCIES/SKILLS NEEDED
- Knowledge of evidence-based approaches to pain management
- Excellent assessment and communication skills
- Strong leadership and organization skills, as rheumatology nurses could assume managerial responsibilities when working in ambulatory centers
- Excellent technical nursing skills such as phlebotomy skills

RELATED WEB SITES AND PROFESSIONAL ORGANIZATIONS
- Rheumatology Nurses Society (http://www.rns-network.org/)
- Arthritis Foundation (http://www.arthritis.org/)
- American College of Rheumatology (http://www.rheumatology.org/)

173 ■ RISK-MANAGEMENT NURSE

BASIC DESCRIPTION
Risk-management nurses have special knowledge and interest in the work environment of nurses and the injuries nurses sustain as a result of environmental exposures. They may be consultants responsible for reviewing medical records, policies, and procedures, and thus would be aware of legal aspects and their implications. Risk-management nurses conduct programs covering the aspects of documentation and internal procedures in order to protect patients and staff from injuries.

EDUCATIONAL REQUIREMENTS
Registered nurse preparation is required.

CORE COMPETENCIES/SKILLS NEEDED
Ability to provide objective view of environment in relation to patient and nurse safety

- Computer skills
- Analytical skills
- Communication skills
- Ability to handle multiple tasks simultaneously
- Sharp visual acuity
- Keen judgement
- Excellent observational skills
- Strong assessment skills

RELATED WEB SITES AND PROFESSIONAL ORGANIZATIONS
- Agency for Health Care Research Quality (www.ahrq.gov)
- Joint Commission for Accreditation of Health Care Organizations (www.jcaho.org)
- American Nurses Association (www.ana.org)

174 ■ RURAL HEALTH NURSE

BASIC DESCRIPTION

A rural health nurse is a generalist who practices professional nursing in communities with relatively low populations that are geographically and often culturally isolated. Rural nurses have close ties to and interaction with the communities in which they practice and often practice with a great deal of autonomy and independence. A strong and varied experience base is crucial in rural nursing, as the population that the rural nurse must care for ranges from infants to the elderly. Therefore, a rural nurse must know about every stage of life. Experience with rural communities is a benefit in order to understand the cultural context within which the people live. For most rural nurses, traveling between isolated communities is part of their role. Rural nurses may operate from a clinic or small hospital, while others may base themselves out of a large mobile health center.

EDUCATIONAL REQUIREMENTS

Registered nurse preparation is required.

CORE COMPETENCIES/SKILLS NEEDED

- Physical assessment and emergency/trauma management skills are vital to the practice for a rural nurse
- Skilled in all areas of nursing, with clinical and assessment skills that reflect this proficiency
- Critical-care skills
- An aptitude for teaching
- A wide knowledge of resources within the community
- Management skills
- Surgical, obstetric, and intravenous therapy skills and the ability to operate and troubleshoot equipment are other useful skills
- Knowledge about the areas such as pharmaceuticals, the region in which one is practicing, as well as an in-depth awareness of cultural norms and values

- Ability to adapt to the resources that are available
- Ability to use innovative and creative solutions to the challenges that exist in locations without major medical centers
- Ability to practice independently, even without the supplies and equipment available that one needs
- Value the close interaction they have with the individuals, families, and communities they serve

RELATED WEB SITE AND PROFESSIONAL ORGANIZATION
- Rural Nursing Organization (www.rno.org)

175 ■ SCHOOL NURSE

BASIC DESCRIPTION
The school nurse practices professional nursing within an educational setting with the goal of assisting students to develop to their greatest physical, emotional, and intellectual ability. School nurses promote health and safety practices and provide interventions to actual and potential health problems. These nurses respond to acute injuries within the school population, as well as assist students to manage chronic conditions, such as food allergies, asthma, and other illnesses. Practice settings include school systems, state health departments, and county health departments.

EDUCATIONAL REQUIREMENTS
Registered nurse preparation is required. Some school systems and/or health departments are requiring that school nurses have baccalaureate or master's degrees in nursing. Certification is available from the National Board for Certification of School Nurses.

CORE COMPETENCIES/SKILLS NEEDED
- General experience with children
- Strong foundation in physical assessment and first aid and emergency care
- A solid skill base and understanding of pediatric medicine
- Knowledge of developmental stages is very important in order to provide age-appropriate care
- Strong communication and interpersonal skills to assess and determine the health care needs of the children and their families
- Computer skills to chart and track students' records and immunization status
- Ability to relate to children and communicate with patients and the school community

- Ability to provide health education
- Responsible for medication management of children while they are in school
- Skills to participate as a member of a multidisciplinary education team and collaborate with other members of the educational environment
- Ability to provide care for minor ailments such as a scraped knee as well as potentially serious conditions such as an allergic reaction or a major injury
- Ensure the safety and well-being of all the children in the school
- Ability to deal with issues such as school violence, suicide, and unwanted teen pregnancies

RELATED WEB SITES AND PROFESSIONAL ORGANIZATIONS

- National Association of School Nurses (www.nasn.org)
- The Association of School Nurses of Connecticut (http://schoolnurse.vservers.com)
- National Association of State School Nurse Consultants (http://www.nassnc.org/)
- National Board for Certification of School Nurses (www.nbcsn.org)

176 ■ SCRUB NURSE

BASIC DESCRIPTION

The scrub nurse is part of the perioperative surgical team who works side by side with the surgeon during the intraoperative phase. The scrub nurse observes strict aseptic technique while providing and anticipating the need for sterile surgical equipment such as scalpels, forceps, and sponges that the surgeon needs during the procedure.

EDUCATIONAL REQUIREMENTS

Registered nurse preparation is highly preferred; Basic Life Support certification is required.

CORE COMPETENCIES/SKILLS NEEDED

- ■ Excellent communication skills
- ■ Ability to anticipate the needs of the surgeon
- ■ Knowledge of surgical asepsis

RELATED WEB SITE AND PROFESSIONAL ORGANIZATION

- ■ Association of Operating Room Nurses (www.aorn.org)

177 ■ SIMULATION LABORATORY DIRECTOR

BASIC DESCRIPTION

A simulation education director works in an academic setting and is responsible for managing daily simulation lab operations, designing and evaluating simulation cases based on educational principles, ensuring growth of the simulation program, updating programs/cases based on latest evidence, and conducting evaluation of the simulation program based on school and professional standard outcomes.

EDUCATIONAL REQUIREMENTS

Master's degree or higher is required; experience as a nurse educator is highly preferred.

CORE COMPETENCIES/SKILLS NEEDED

- Knowledge of budgeting and accounting, technology and simulation software, equipment being used, quality improvement, regulations, and regulatory guidelines (patient safety guidelines)
- Excellent organization, communication, leadership, and interpersonal skills
- Knowledge of adult learning principles
- Strong clinical skills

RELATED WEB SITES AND PROFESSIONAL ORGANIZATIONS

- International Nursing Association for Clinical Nursing Simulation (http://www.inacsl.org/INACSL_2010/index.php)
- National League for Nursing Simulation Innovation Resource Center (http://sirc.nln.org/)

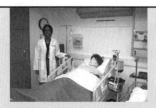

Profile:
KELLI BRYANT
Simulation Laboratory Director

1. What is your educational background in nursing (and other areas) and what formal credentials do you hold?

I received my associate and bachelor's degree in nursing. I continued my education and received a master's degree is nursing majoring as a women's health nurse practitioner. Recently I received a professional doctorate, a Doctorate of Nursing Practice degree with a focus on nursing education. I am a board-certified Women's Health Nurse Practitioner and Certified Childbirth Educator. I also have a certificate in simulation.

2. How did you first become interested in the career that you are currently in?

My interest in simulation was sparked by a demonstration of SimMan Laerdal and Birthing Noelle Gaumard patient simulators. I have always been a person who loves technological gadgets and working with computers. About a year after I was introduced to simulation, a colleague recommended me for a part-time position at her institution as a simulation coordinator. The college received a grant to implement simulation and was looking for a part-time simulation coordinator to implement simulation into the nursing curriculum. I accepted the position and successfully implemented simulation into each medical–surgical course. After working as a professor full time for 7 years and working as a simulation lab coordinator part-time, I decided to pursue a full-time job in simulation. Fortunately, I was hired as a director of simulation learning at a major university. I currently coordinate and implement over 40 simulation sessions a week for the undergraduate and graduate nursing programs. Simulation has allowed me the opportunity to teach faculty and students while still permitting me to use my creativity to create realistic clinical experiences for students.

Continued

177 ■ Simulation Laboratory Director

Profile: KELLI BRYANT Continued

3. What are the most rewarding aspects of your career?

My job is exciting, innovative, and challenging. I enjoy running and programming all of our high-tech patient manikins and creating realistic patient scenarios using trained actors. Simulation is the wave of the future in nursing education, and I enjoy being in the forefront of the science of simulation learning. In the past year I have had visitors from South Africa, Australia, China, and Israel who have come to the Simulation Learning Center in order to gain knowledge in simulation. I take pleasure in becoming an expert in my field and sharing my knowledge with other nursing faculty throughout the world.

4. What advice would you give to someone contemplating the same career path in nursing?

I would encourage anyone interested in simulation to expand their knowledge about simulation by attending conferences, reading journal articles, and obtaining simulation training. Individuals interested in simulation should join simulation organizations such as International Nursing Association for Clinical Simulation and Learning and the Society for Simulation in Healthcare where they can network with other simulation experts. I would also encourage interested individuals to receive simulation training, which is offered through patient simulator companies or organizations such as National League of Nursing and Drexel University.

178 ■ SPACE NURSE/ASTRONAUT

BASIC DESCRIPTION

Space nurses provide on-the-ground monitoring and a full range of health services to more than 400 astronauts, who are screened to determine if they meet the National Aeronautics and Space Administration (NASA) health requirements and, in some cases, military stipulations. These data must be meticulously documented, because they are used to follow the health of astronauts throughout their lifetimes and to determine service eligibility, and are crucial to mission safety. Flight medicine clinic nurses also coordinate dietary and fitness services; clinic nurses staff a "sick call" service for astronauts to use before and after flight. At the first sign of physical discomfort, an astronaut first contacts a nurse, who administers appropriate treatment. Other nurses are employed as support staff for proctology and cardiovascular clinics and as instructors on the basis of self-assessment and medication administration for astronauts. Space Nurse Society members now meet at yearly conferences to exchange ideas, share research findings, and discuss the application of nursing methods used on Earth in space settings. Many members are nurse researchers who study the health risks associated with space travel.

EDUCATIONAL REQUIREMENTS

Registered nurse preparation is required; graduate preparation is required for researchers.

CORE COMPETENCIES/SKILLS NEEDED

- Excellent assessment skills
- Interest in, and knowledge of, aerospace industry and challenges
- Mental health skills
- Innovation and creativity
- Knowledge of physics and engineering

RELATED WEB SITES AND PROFESSIONAL ORGANIZATIONS

- The Space Nursing Society (www.geocities.com/spacenursingsociety/)
- The Mars Society (www.marssociety.org)
- NASA Headquarters (www.nasa.gov)
- NASA jobs (www.nasajobs.nasa.gov)

179 ■ SPINAL CORD INJURY NURSE

BASIC DESCRIPTION
Spinal cord injury (SCI) nurses play a vital role in maintaining the patient's respiratory, gastrointestinal, urinary, musculoskeletal, and integumentary systems and in providing psychological support to the patient and family. Caring for a patient with an SCI is complex and demanding. Although the primary focus in acute care management is directed toward sustaining life, it is critical that nurses involved in acute care management realize the effect their care has on the patient's rehabilitation and future life. By working to avoid preventable complications that cause additional morbidity and delay rehabilitation, nurses in acute care settings can help people with this devastating injury have the best possible opportunity to regain their health.

EDUCATIONAL REQUIREMENTS
Registered nurse preparation is required.

CORE COMPETENCIES/SKILLS NEEDED
- Excellent clinical skills
- Team skills for collaboration with respiratory and physical therapy to protect respiratory function
- Knowledge of the rehabilitation processes used in provision of care
- Good interpersonal skills
- Skills in helping patients and families manage anxiety by providing them with accurate information about the consequences of the injury in terms they can understand and by offering realistic hope for the future

RELATED WEB SITES AND PROFESSIONAL ORGANIZATIONS
- American Spinal Injury Association (www.asia-spinalinjury.org/index.html)
- Spinal Cord Injury: The Acute Phase (two-part series), by Maureen Habel, MA, RN (www.nurseweek.com/ce/ce107a.asp#ref)

180 ■ STAFF DEVELOPMENT EDUCATOR

BASIC DESCRIPTION

The staff development educator incorporates a variety of roles into the teaching of new staff members. They are responsible for the basic orientation and continuing education for new nurses and nursing staff employed by hospitals and other health care organizations. They monitor the overall staff compliance with clinical performance standards and participate in providing ongoing continuing education for nursing staff. They may specialize in certain clinical areas (e.g., gerontology, oncology) or they may be generalists. These educators function in a number of settings including hospitals, senior centers, clinics, health maintenance organizations, and schools of nursing.

EDUCATIONAL REQUIREMENTS

Registered nurse preparation is required; Bachelor of Science in Nursing or Master of Science in Nursing is preferred in some settings. Certification on Nursing Professional Development is available from the American Nurses Credentialing Center.

CORE COMPETENCIES/SKILLS NEEDED

- Ability to set priorities
- Knowledge of adult learning theory
- Ability to be an effective teacher
- Excellent communication skills
- Commitment to lifelong learning
- Ability to develop and implement lesson plans
- Staff development experience
- Positive attitude and enthusiasm for learning
- Ability to manage time effectively
- Ability to function autonomously

RELATED WEB SITES AND PROFESSIONAL ORGANIZATIONS

- National Nursing Staff Development Organization (www.nnsdo.org)
- American Nurses Credentialing Center (ww.nursecredentialing.org)

181 ■ STAFF NURSE

BASIC DESCRIPTION

A staff nurse is a generalized job description of someone who works in a health care setting or facility. She/he works side by side with members of the health care team to treat and manage patients' conditions across age groups. Staff nurses' responsibilities are outlined by the employer.

EDUCATIONAL REQUIREMENTS

Registered nurse preparation; Bachelor of Science in Nursing are highly preferred.

CORE COMPETENCIES/SKILLS NEEDED

- Excellent communication and interpersonal skills
- Advanced knowledge required based on area of specialization
- Knowledge of scope of nursing practice defined by state board of nursing

RELATED WEB SITE AND PROFESSIONAL ORGANIZATION

- State board of nursing

182 ■ SUBACUTE/TRANSITION CARE NURSE

BASIC DESCRIPTION
Subacute or transition care nurses care for patients who have skilled care needs after an acute illness or hospitalization. Care could be rendered in a rehabilitation or skilled nursing facility or in a designated unit of a health care facility.

EDUCATIONAL REQUIREMENTS
Registered nurse preparation and Basic Life Support certification are required.

CORE COMPETENCIES/SKILLS NEEDED
- Medical and surgical nursing experience
- Excellent assessment skills, and skill in the care of patients on intravenous therapy, ventilator, or tracheostomy
- Strong computer and documentation skills
- Ability to solve staffing difficulties when they arise
- Ability to work in a dynamic unit where patient admission and discharges are high

RELATED WEB SITE AND PROFESSIONAL ORGANIZATION
- American Subacute Care Association

183 ■ TELEHEALTH NURSE

BASIC DESCRIPTION
A telehealth nurse conducts patient assessment, education, crisis intervention, counseling, and triage over the telephone or other forms of interactive media. They utilize care protocols, standards, and guidelines in arriving at decisions. They could be employed by home care agencies or insurance and medical groups.

EDUCATIONAL REQUIREMENTS
A registered nurse license is required; certification in telehealth nursing as part of ambulatory nursing is provided by the American Academy of Ambulatory Care Nursing.

CORE COMPETENCIES/SKILLS NEEDED
- Good communication skills
- Ability to sit for long periods
- Strong computer skills and ability to comfortably use computer-based guidelines
- Strong documentation skills using the electronic health/documentation record

RELATED WEB SITE AND PROFESSIONAL ORGANIZATION
- American Academy of Ambulatory Care Nursing (www.aaacn.org)

184 ■ TELEMETRY NURSE

BASIC DESCRIPTION
Telemetry nurses assess acute changes in patients and work in a fast-paced environment. These nurses monitor the heart rhythm of patients in special care units of hospitals and analyze heart rhythms, interpret ECGs, note arrhythmias, and intervene in emergency situations.

EDUCATIONAL REQUIREMENTS
Registered nurse preparation is required. Certification as Progressive Care Certified Nurse is available from the American Association of Critical Care Nurses Certification Corporation.

CORE COMPETENCIES/SKILLS NEEDED
- Excellent clinical skills
- Critical thinking ability
- Cardiovascular knowledge, including anatomy and physiology and cardiac disease processes
- Skill in patient teaching about medications, dietary changes, and post-myocardial infarction activity restrictions
- Flexibility given the unpredictability of the patient status
- Ability to use technology available for patient monitoring

RELATED WEB SITE AND PROFESSIONAL ORGANIZATION
- American Association of Critical Care Nurses Certification Corporation (www.cetcorp.org)

185 ■ TELEPHONIC TRIAGE NURSE

BASIC DESCRIPTION

A telephone triage nurse provides a variety of services and information to patients over the phone. Most often, they are using written protocols to guide their practice and are determining the urgency of care needed and scheduling appointments or directing callers to health care providers as needed. Accordingly, the goal of this unique form of nursing is to decrease unnecessary visits to physicians, nurse practitioners, and the emergency room as well as to provide information for self-care. Some triage nurses working for medical practices or clinics may be familiar with the patient and their health status. More often, though, the nurse must use his or her excellent communication and information-gathering skills to determine the best course of action for the patient. Triage nurses deal with the entire spectrum, from healthy patients to the acute and chronically ill. Triage nurses usually have regular hours but there is no direct patient contact, and triage nurses may spend long hours at a desk on the telephone and computer. There are opportunities to work in a variety of settings such as medical offices, health maintenance organizations, insurance companies, hospitals, clinics, and triage centers.

EDUCATIONAL REQUIREMENTS

Registered nurse preparation and Bachelor of Science in Nursing are preferred. Previous emergency department or triage experience is highly desired for this role; Advanced Cardiac Life Support and Basic Life Support certifications are often required. Employers may require completion of Telehealth Nursing Practice Core Course.

CORE COMPETENCIES/SKILLS NEEDED

■ Previous experience with triage, either on the telephone or in an emergency room
■ Critical thinking skills

■ Ability to determine the problem within the first few sentences of a conversation; a certain intuitive ability can be useful in assessing the situation and making the correct decision for the patient
■ Superior verbal communication skills are essential
■ Strong assessment skills
■ Excellent clinical skills
■ Crisis intervention skills
■ Typing and computer ability to keep track of information gathered during the telephone conversation
■ Teaching ability, as patients may require instruction for self-care and/or symptom management
■ Ability to remain calm in high-stress situations

RELATED WEB SITES AND PROFESSIONAL ORGANIZATIONS

■ All Health Net: Telephone Triage Nursing (www.allhealthnet.com/Nursing/Telephone+Triage/)
■ Information about Telephone Triage for Nurses (www.geocities.com/hanson1517/nursesinformationpage.html)
■ International Telenurses Association (www.intellinurse.org)
■ The American Academy of Ambulatory Care Nursing (www.aaacn.org)

186 ■ TRANSCULTURAL NURSE

BASIC DESCRIPTION
This advanced registered nurse's role aims to expertly promote and provide culturally competent and congruent care to individuals, groups, and communities. This title also entails expertise in providing quality care based on transcultural nursing practices by transcultural nursing scholars.

EDUCATIONAL REQUIREMENTS
A registered nurse license is required; educational preparation at the master's, postmaster's, or doctoral level is required for certification along with completion of one 3-credit course on cultural diversity or competence, 2,400 hours in transcultural nursing clinical practice, research, or teaching.

CORE COMPETENCIES/SKILLS NEEDED
- Ability to provide culturally sensitive and congruent care to diverse patient populations
- Knowledge of transcultural nursing theories and their applications
- Excellent communication skills
- Ability to work in a team

RELATED WEB SITES AND PROFESSIONAL ORGANIZATIONS
- Transcultural Nursing Society (www.tcns.org)
- American Association of Colleges of Nursing Cultural Competency Web site (http://www.aacn.nche.edu/Education/cultural.htm)

187 ■ TRANSPLANT NURSE

BASIC DESCRIPTION
The transplant nurse cares for recipient and living-donor patients through-out the transplantation process from end-stage disease processes to the preoperative, operative, and postoperative care. The transplant nurse is most often employed by the hospital with a transplant center. Practice roles can include nurse practitioner, case manager, transplant coordina-tor, research nurse, organ procurement nurse, and clinical specialist.

EDUCATIONAL REQUIREMENTS
Registered nurse preparation is required; Bachelor of Science in Nursing or Master of Science in Nursing is often preferred.

CORE COMPETENCIES/SKILLS NEEDED
- Knowledge of transplant processes
- Excellent communication skills
- Teaching skills
- Knowledge of high-tech treatments
- Sensitivity in dealing with emotional and ethical issues
- Technological skills
- Ability to work with interdisciplinary team

RELATED WEB SITES AND PROFESSIONAL ORGANIZATIONS
- International Transplant Nurses Society (www.itns.org/)
- International Society for Heart and Lung Transplantation (www.ishlt.org/)

188 ■ TRAUMA NURSE

BASIC DESCRIPTION
A trauma nurse cares for patients who have multisystem trauma across all age groups and works in acute care facilities and transport units.

EDUCATIONAL REQUIREMENTS
Registered nurse license and Bachelor of Science in Nursing are preferred; Advanced Cardiac Life Support, Basic Life Support, Pediatric Advanced Life Support, and Trauma Course certifications are required; certification is offered by the Emergency Nurses Association.

CORE COMPETENCIES/SKILLS NEEDED
- Excellent clinical, critical thinking, and decision-making skills
- Knowledge of critical care and emergency medicine concepts across all age groups
- Ability to work in a dynamic high-stress environment
- Flexible, motivated, and excellent communication and interpersonal skills
- Team player and excellent organizational skills

RELATED WEB SITE AND PROFESSIONAL ORGANIZATION
- Emergency Nurses Association (www.ena.org)

189 ■ TRAVEL NURSE

BASIC DESCRIPTION

Travel nurses are those who travel and take temporary nursing assignments, usually lasting 8 to 26 weeks (average is 13 weeks), in locations of the nurse's choice, in facilities across the United States and internationally. Travel nurses often work in hospital settings in staff nurse positions, but may also be found on cruise ships, in rural settings, or other roles that require the skill of a registered nurse. A travel nurse works with an agency that makes arrangements for the position, provides accommodations at the location, and pays for travel expenses. The work activities depend on the location and the type of assignment. A nurse could go from a tertiary intensive care unit, caring for a postoperative coronary bypass patient, to a small 30-bed hospital where nurses care for a child with pneumonia next to an elderly patient with a stroke. Travel nurses are those who thrive on diversity and enjoy the opportunity to travel and experience new places and cultures.

EDUCATIONAL REQUIREMENTS

Registered nurse preparation is required; experience as a nurse is often preferred but not required.

CORE COMPETENCIES/SKILLS NEEDED

- Strong clinical skills; a critical care background is highly recommended, but not required
- Flexibility and adaptability
- Strong communication skills and the ability to get along with people to help integration within a unit and foster positive working relationships
- Adaptable to change

RELATED WEB SITES AND PROFESSIONAL ORGANIZATIONS

- National Association of Traveling Nurses (www.travelingnurse.org)
- NursesRx (www.nursesrx.com)
- Preferred Healthcare Staffing (www.preferredhealthcare.com)
- TravelNursing.com (www.travelnurse.com)
- PSR Nurses (www.psrnurses.com)

190 ■ TRIAGE NURSE

BASIC DESCRIPTION

A triage nurse is a specialized emergency department (ED) nursing role that is responsible for conducting a focused assessment and prioritizing a patient's clinical condition for the purpose of providing immediate care if the patient requires it. Although the triage nurse does not usually provide immediate care, she may be required to deliver hands-on care if the situation calls for it.

EDUCATIONAL REQUIREMENTS

Active registered nurse license and Bachelor of Science in Nursing are preferred. Previous ED or triage experience is highly desired for this role; Advanced Cardiac Life Support and Basic Life Support certifications are required.

CORE COMPETENCIES/SKILLS NEEDED

- Excellent assessment and problem-solving skills
- Ability to perform in high-stress situation that calls for quick thinking and analysis
- Good communication skills

RELATED WEB SITES AND PROFESSIONAL ORGANIZATIONS

- Emergency Nurses Association (www.ena.org)
- Association of Critical Nurses Association (www.aacn.org)

191 ■ UNDERWRITER NURSE

BASIC DESCRIPTION

An underwriter nurse is responsible for assessing a patient's medical and insurance risks. Also, their medical and nursing backgrounds allow them to serve as consultants to help insurance agents arrive at a patient's medical risk.

EDUCATIONAL REQUIREMENTS

Registered nurse preparation is required, and most positions require a Bachelor of Science in Nursing.

CORE COMPETENCIES/SKILLS NEEDED

- Good computer skills
- Excellent interpersonal and communication skills
- Excellent decision-making skills
- Thorough knowledge of health insurance industry

RELATED WEB SITE AND PROFESSIONAL ORGANIZATION

- Group Underwriters Association of America (http://www.guaa.com/)

192 ■ UNIVERSITY PROVOST/PRESIDENT

BASIC DESCRIPTION
The university provost or president leads the faculty in fostering excellent teaching and ensuring sound scholarship, clinical expertise, and research. The university president or provost articulates the vision of the university or school through leadership in school, university, and professional activities.

EDUCATIONAL REQUIREMENTS
PhD or EdD preparation is required.

CORE COMPETENCIES/SKILLS NEEDED
- Proven record of administrative leadership
- Experience in teaching nursing at a college or university level
- Grant writing and/or research funding skills and experience
- Scholarly publications
- Record of service to the community/profession commensurate with the rank of associate or full professor
- Excellent interpersonal skills
- Motivation (high energy)
- Ability to work with others
- Creativity
- Leadership

RELATED WEB SITES AND PROFESSIONAL ORGANIZATIONS
- Sigma Theta Tau Honor Society of Nursing (www.nursingsociety.org)
- American Nurses Credentialing Center (www.nursingworld.org/ancc/index.htm)

193 ■ UROLOGY NURSE

BASIC DESCRIPTION
A urology nurse specializes in the care of patients who have urologic conditions such as kidney stones, urinary tract infections, and cancers. They work in either inpatient or outpatient units. Aside from providing direct care, they also educate patients on preventing recurrences of acute conditions and avoiding complications.

EDUCATIONAL REQUIREMENTS
Registered nurse license and Basic Life Support certification are required; Bachelor of Science in Nursing is highly preferred; certification is offered by the Certification Board for Urologic Nurses.

CORE COMPETENCIES/SKILLS NEEDED
- Must possess a solid knowledge of the male and female urinary tract and reproductive systems, pathophysiology, and treatments
- Excellent bedside manners and sensitivity
- Strong computer and documentation skills

RELATED WEB SITES AND PROFESSIONAL ORGANIZATIONS
- Society of Urologic Nurses and Associates (www.suna.org)
- American Urological Association (www.aua.org)
- The Global Alliance of Urology Nurses (www.thegaun.org)
- National Association for Continence (www.nafc.org)

194 ■ UTILIZATION REVIEW NURSE

BASIC DESCRIPTION
A utilization review (UR) nurse reviews and makes decisions about the appropriateness and level of patient care being provided. The eventual goal of UR nurses is to provide cost-effective care and ensure proper utilization of resources.

EDUCATIONAL REQUIREMENTS
Registered nurse preparation is required; Bachelor of Science in Nursing is required in most positions; certification in health care quality and management is offered by the American Board of Quality Assurance and Utilization Review Physicians, Inc.

CORE COMPETENCIES/SKILLS NEEDED
- Ability to work under stress and with autonomy
- Excellent organization and leadership skills
- Excellent interpersonal and communication skills
- Experience in case management is highly desirable

RELATED WEB SITE AND PROFESSIONAL ORGANIZATION
- American Board of Quality Assurance and Utilization Review Physicians, Inc. (http://www.abqaurp.org/whoshould.asp)

195 ■ VACCINATION NURSE

BASIC DESCRIPTION
The vaccination or immunization nurse is responsible for providing vaccination to clients across age groups based on immunization guidelines and schedules, and federal, state, or county protocols.

EDUCATIONAL REQUIREMENTS
A registered nurse license is highly preferred in most states; Basic Life Support certification is required.

CORE COMPETENCIES/SKILLS NEEDED
- Knowledge of vaccines–immunization schedule, correct anatomical sites, correct dosage, indications, contraindications, side effects, and steps to be taken during an anaphylactic reaction
- Knowledge of infection-control practices
- Excellent communication and customer service orientation skills

RELATED WEB SITES AND PROFESSIONAL ORGANIZATIONS
- State department of health
- American Nurses Association (www.nursingworld.org)

196 ■ VASCULAR NURSE

BASIC DESCRIPTION
The vascular nurse is responsible for nursing care of patients who have chronic vascular diseases mostly seen in outpatient medical offices. A vascular nurse's job responsibility could include assisting the physician with treatment, minor surgical procedures, and administering medications.

EDUCATIONAL REQUIREMENTS
Registered nurse license is preferred; Basic Life Support certification is required for most positions; experience in medical–surgical unit or critical care is highly desirable; certification as cardiac vascular nurse is offered by the American Nurses Credentialing Center

CORE COMPETENCIES/SKILLS NEEDED
- Astute assessment skills
- Excellent communication and interpersonal skills
- Good organizational and managerial skills as the job may include administrative responsibilities in the vascular clinic
- Computer literacy is required

RELATED WEB SITES AND PROFESSIONAL ORGANIZATIONS
- American Nurses Credentialing Center (www.nursecredentialing.org)
- Society for Vascular Nursing (www.svnnet.org)

197 ■ VETERINARIAN NURSE

BASIC DESCRIPTION
A veterinary nurse works alongside a veterinarian in caring for animals. Their job responsibilities vary from administering medications to treating wounds, performing tests, and conducting home pet visits. Areas of employment include animal laboratories, zoos, and organizations that protect the welfare of animals like the American Society for the Prevention of Cruelty to Animals.

EDUCATIONAL REQUIREMENTS
Registered nurse preparation is preferred.

CORE COMPETENCIES/SKILLS NEEDED
- Knowledge related to pet health
- Ability to work with members of the veterinary team
- Strong organizational skills as the job may also involve managerial responsibilities
- Strong intravenous skills

RELATED WEB SITE AND PROFESSIONAL ORGANIZATION
- American Society for the Prevention of Cruelty to Animals (http://www.aspca.org/)

198 ■ WOMEN'S HEALTH NURSE

BASIC DESCRIPTION
Women's health practitioners focus on primary care for women across the life span, from adolescence to the elderly. They may be prepared for basic nursing positions or as advanced practice nurses and provide services in hospitals and a range of primary care and community-based settings.

EDUCATIONAL REQUIREMENTS
Registered nurse preparation or advanced practice certification is required. Certification in various specialized women's health and primary care nursing is available from the National Certification Corporation for the Obstetric, Gynecological, and Neonatal Nursing Specialties.

CORE COMPETENCIES/SKILLS NEEDED
- Ability to perform well-woman assessments
- Instruction in self-breast examinations and breast health education
- Knowledge of women's health
- Patient education
- Ability to provide care to women across populations, social classes, and socioeconomic and age groups, and in urban, suburban, and rural settings

RELATED WEB SITES AND PROFESSIONAL ORGANIZATIONS
- National Association for Women's Health (www.nawh.org)
- Association of Women's Health, Obstetric and Neonatal Nurses (www.awhonn.org)
- National Association of Nurse Practitioners in Women's Health (www.npwh.org)
- National Certification Corporation for the Obstetric, Gynecological, and Neonatal Nursing Specialties (www.nccwebsite.org)

199 ■ WOMEN'S HEALTH NURSE PRACTITIONER

BASIC DESCRIPTION
Working with women at different age groups, women's health nurse practitioners provide primary care for women who have gynecological, obstetrical, and family planning needs or issues. They also provide health education and counseling on issues that relate to women's health.

EDUCATIONAL REQUIREMENTS
Registered nurse preparation, Nurse Practitioner certification, and Basic Life Support certification are required; certification is offered by the National Certification Corporation.

CORE COMPETENCIES/SKILLS NEEDED
- Advanced knowledge that relates to obstetrical/gynecological assessment, pathophysiology, and its associated disease management
- Knowledge of unique needs of women
- Excellent communication and interpersonal skills
- Strong computer skills
- Strong organizational and leadership skills

RELATED WEB SITES AND PROFESSIONAL ORGANIZATIONS
- Nurse Practitioners in Women's Health (http://www.npwh.org/i4a/pages/index.cfm?pageid=1)
- American Academy of Nurse Practitioners (http://www.aanp.org/AANPCMS2)
- National Certification Corporation (www.nccwebsite.org)

200 ■ WOUND/OSTOMY/CONTINENCE NURSE

BASIC DESCRIPTION

A wound/ostomy/continence nurse is a registered nurse specializing in the care of skin, particularly involving wounds, healing, and ostomy care and appliances. Hospitals and long-term care facilities employ most of the nurses, and some work in home care.

EDUCATIONAL REQUIREMENTS

Registered nurse preparation is required. Certification is available through the Wound Ostomy Continence Nursing Certification Board.

CORE COMPETENCIES/SKILLS NEEDED

- Excellent aseptic technique
- Excellent wound assessment skills and abilities, and wound care techniques
- Special knowledge of wound healing and skin physiology
- Ability to work independently and with a team
- Excellent documentation skills
- Knowledge of products, appliances, and wound healing
- Responsible for dressing changes, assessment, selection of appropriate appliances, and topical wound healing, as well as pharmacological preparations
- Skill in teaching wound care and maintenance to other staff and patients
- Ability to maintain and promote ostomy care and teach patients to monitor their own appliances
- Skill in patient, family, and staff education
- Photographic documentation

RELATED WEB SITES AND PROFESSIONAL ORGANIZATIONS

- Wound, Ostomy and Continence Nurses Society (www.wocn.org)
- Wound Ostomy Continence Nursing Certification Board (www.wocncb.org/)

201 ■ WOUND OSTOMY CONTINENCE CARE NURSE PRACTITIONER

BASIC DESCRIPTION

The wound ostomy care nurse practitioner provides primary care to patients requiring ostomy and wound care that includes accurate assessment, documentation, treatment, and evaluation of care based on national standards and evidence-based guidelines. Aside from providing clinical services, the wound ostomy continence care nurse practitioner is also involved in patient teaching and care coordination to ensure timely recovery and discharge and serves as a consultant to institution and community partner organizations.

EDUCATIONAL REQUIREMENTS

Registered nurse (RN) preparation and Nurse Practitioner (NP) certification are required; most job positions require a 1-year experience as an NP and 5 years experience as an RN; certification is available from the Wound Ostomy and Continence Nursing Certification Board.

CORE COMPETENCIES/SKILLS NEEDED

- Excellent assessment, interpersonal, and critical analysis skills
- Sensitivity to the needs of patients and their families
- Ability to work in a team
- Strong leadership and organizational skills
- Strong computer and documentation skills

RELATED WEB SITES AND PROFESSIONAL ORGANIZATIONS

- Wound Ostomy and Continence Nursing Certification Board (http://www.wocncb.org/become-certified/advanced-practice/)
- Wound Ostomy and Continence Nurses Society (http://www.wocncb.org/become-certified/advanced-practice/)

◼ APPENDICES

■ APPENDIX A: YOUR GUIDE TO CERTIFICATION

For a more detailed chart of the eligibility requirements and fees go to www.nursingcenter.com/ajncareerguide2008.

AMERICAN NURSES CREDENTIALING CENTER (ANCC)
8515 Georgia Avenue, Suite 400 Silver Spring, MD 20910-3492 (800) 284-2378
www.nursecredentialing.org

Credentials: Acute Care Nurse Practitioner **(APRN,BC*)**; Adult Health Clinical Nurse Specialist **(APRN,BC*)**; Adult Nurse Practitioner **(APRN,BC*)**; Adult Psychiatric & Mental Health Clinical Nurse Specialist **(APRN,BC*)**; Adult Psychiatric & Mental Health Nurse Practitioner **(APRN,BC*)**; Ambulatory Care Nursing **(RN-BC†)**; Cardiac Vascular Nursing **(RN-BC†)**; Case Management Nursing **(RN-BC†)**; Child/Adolescent Psychiatric & Mental Health Clinical Nurse Specialist **(APRN,BC*)**; Diabetes Management, Advanced **(APRN,BC-ADM*)** or **(RPh,BC-ADM*)** or **(RD,BC-ADM*)**; Family Nurse Practitioner **(APRN,BC*)**; Family Psychiatric & Mental Health Nurse Practitioner **(APRN,BC*)**; Gerontology Clinical Nurse Specialist **(APRN,BC*)**; Gerontological Nursing **(RN-BC†)**; Gerontological Nurse Practitioner **(APRN,BC*)**; Informatics **(RN-BC†)**; Medical-Surgical Nursing **(RN-BC1)**; Nursing Administration **(CNA,BC†)**; Nursing Administration, Advanced **(CNAA,BC*)**; Nursing Professional Development **(RN-BC†)**; Pain Management **(RN-BC†)**; Pediatrics Clinical Nurse Specialist **(APRN,BC*)**; Pediatric Nursing **(RN-BC†)**; Pediatric Nurse Practitioner **(APRN,BC*)**; Psychiatric & Mental Health Nursing **(RN-BC†)**; Public/Community Health Clinical Nurse Specialist **(APRN,BC*)**

ACADEMIC NURSE EDUCATOR
National League for Nursing
61 Broadway, 33rd Floor
New York, NY 10006
(800) 669-1656
www.nln.org/FacultyCertification/index.htm

Credential: (CNE)

ADDICTIONS NURSING
CARN Certification
International Nurses Society on Addictions
P.O. Box 163635
Columbus, OH 43216
(614) 221-9989
Fax:(614) 221-2335
intnsa@intnsa.org
www.intnsa.org

Credentials: (CARN); (CARN-AP)

CHILDBIRTH EDUCATORS
Lamaze International
2025 M St., NW, Suite 800
Washington, DC 20036
(800) 368-4404
www.lamaze.org

Credential: (LCCE†)

---

* Will change mid-2008
† Formerly RN,BC
‡ Formerly ACCE
§ Has met the standards of the American Board of Nursing Specialties, a national peer review program.
ǁ See also the offerings of the ANCC.

CRITICAL CARE NURSING[||]
AACN Certification Corporation
101 Columbia
AlisoViejo, CA 92656-4109
(800) 899-2226; (949) 362-2000
certcorp@aacn.org
www.certcorp.org

Credentials: Adult Critical-Care Nurse **(CCRN)**; Cardiac Medicine Certification **(CMC)**; Cardiac Surgery Certification **(CSC)**; Clinical Nurse Specialist in Acute and Critical Care; Adult, Neonatal, or Pediatric **(CCNS)**; Neonatal Critical-Care Nurse **(CCRN)**; Pediatric Critical-Care Nurse **(CCRN)**; Progressive Care Certified Nurse **(PCCN)**

DIABETES EDUCATORS
National Certification Board for
    Diabetes Educators
330 East Algonquin Rd., Suite 4
Arlington Heights, IL 60005
info@ncbde.org
www.ncbde.org

Credential: (CDE)

EMERGENCY NURSING
Board of Certification for Emergency Nursing
915 Lee St. DesPlaines, IL 60016
bcen@ena.org
www.ena.org/bcen

Credential: (CEN)

FLIGHT NURSING
Board of Certification for Emergency Nursing
915 Lee St. DesPlaines, IL60016
bcen@ena.org
www.ena.org/bcen

Credentials: (CFRN); (CTRN)

GASTROENTEROLOGY
American Board of Certification for
    Gastroenterology Nurses, Inc.
401 North Michigan Avenue
Chicago, IL 60611-4267
info@abcgn.org
www.abcgn.org

Credentials: (CGN); (CGRN)

GENETICS NURSING
Genetic Nursing Credentialing Commission, Inc.
P.O. Box 67
Keuka Park, NY 14478
www.geneticnurse.org

Credentials: Advanced Practice Nurse in Genetics **(APNG)**; Genetics Clinical Nurse **(GCN)**

HEALTH CARE QUALITY
Healthcare Quality Certification Board
P.O. Box 19604
Lenexa, KS 66285-9604
info@cphq.org
www.cphq.org

Credential: (CPHQ)

HIV/AIDS NURSING
HIV/AIDS Nursing Certification Board
3538 Ridgewood Road
Akron, OH 44333
www.anacnet.org/certification/ hancb/ index.html

Credentials: AIDS Certified Registered Nurse **(ACRN)**; Advanced AIDS Certified Registered Nurse **(AACRN)**

HOLISTIC NURSING
American Holistic Nurses'
    Certification Corp.
811 Linden Loop
Cedar Park, TX 78613
(877) 284-0998
AHNCC@flash.net
ahncc@flash.net
www.ahncc.org

Credentials: (HN-BC); (AHN-BC)

HOSPICE AND PALLIATIVE NURSING
National Board for Certification of Hospice and
    Palliative Nurses
One Penn Center West One, Suite 229
Pittsburgh, PA 15276
nbchpn@hpna.org
www.nbchpn.org

Credentials: (ACHPN); (CHPN)
(CHPLN); (CHPNA)

INFECTION CONTROL
Certification Board of Infection Control and
    Epidemiology, Inc.
P.O. Box 19554
Lenexa, KS 66285
cbic-info@goAMP.com
www.cbic.org

Credential: (CIC)

INFUSION NURSING

Infusion Nurses Certification
Corporation 315 Norwood Park S.
Norwood, MA 02062
julie.smiley@ins1.org
www.incc1.org

Credential: (CRNI)

LACTATION CONSULTANT

International Board of Lactation
    Consultant Examiners
7245 Arlington Blvd., Suite 300
Falls Church, VA 22042-3215
(703) 560-7330
iblce@iblce.org
www.iblce.org

Credential: (IBCLC)

LEGAL NURSE CONSULTING

American Legal Nurse Consultant
    Certification Board[§]
401 N. Michigan Ave., Suite 2200
Chicago, IL 60611-4267
info@lnccertified.org
www.lnccertified.org

Credential: (LNCC)

MANAGED CARE NURSING

American Board of Managed
    Care Nursing
4435 Waterfront Dr., Suite 101
Glen Allen, VA 23060
keads@abmcn.org
www.abmcn.org

Credential: (CMCN)

MEDICAL-SURGICAL NURSING[‖]

Medical-Surgical Nursing
    Certification Board
MSNCB National Office
East Hol lyAve., P.O. Box 56
Pitman, NJ 08071-0056
msncb@ajj.com
www.medsurgnurse.org

Credential: (CMSRN)

NEPHROLOGY NURSING

Board of Nephrology Examiners Nursing and
    Technology (BONENT)
1901 Pennsylvania Ave. NW Suite 607
Washington, DC 20006
Phone:(202) 462-1252
Fax:(202) 463-1257

peter@bonent.org
www.bonent.org

Credential: (CHN); (CPDN); (CHT)

NEPHROLOGY NURSING CERTIFICATION COMMISSION

East Holly Ave., Box 56
Pitman, NJ 08071-0056
nncc@ajj.com
www.nncc-exam.org

Credentials: (CNN); (CDN); (CCHT)

NEUROSCIENCE NURSING

American Board of Neuroscience Nursing
4700 W. Lake Ave.
Glenview, IL 60025
info@aann.org
www.aann.org

Credential: (CNRN)

NURSE ADMINISTRATION—LONG-TERM CARE

NADONA/LTC Certification Registrar
Reed Hartman Tower,
11353 Reed Hartman Highway, Suite 210
Cincinnati, OH 45241
info@nadona.org
www.nadona.org

Credential: (CDONA/LTC)

NURSE ANESTHETIST

Council on Recertification of Nurse Anesthetists[§]
222 South Prospect Ave.
Park Ridge, IL 60068-5790
recertification@aana.com
www.aana.com/council/default.asp

Credential: (CRNA)

NURSE MIDWIFERY AND MIDWIFERY

American Midwifery Certification Board
849 International Drive, Suite 205
Linthicum, MD 21090
www.amcbmidwife.org

Credentials: (CNM); (CM)

NURSES IN NUTRITION SUPPORT

National Board of Nutrition Support Certification
American Society for Parenteral and Enteral
    Nutrition (ASPEN)
8630 Fenton St., Suite 412
Silver Spring, MD 20910-3805
nbnsc@nutr.org or aspen@nutr.org
www.nutritioncertify.org

Credential: (CNSN)

OCCUPATIONAL HEALTH NURSING
American Board for Occupational
  Health Nurses, Inc.
201 East Ogden, Suite 114
Hinsdale, IL 60521-3652
info@abohn.org
www.abohn.org

Credentials: (COHN[§]); (COHN-S[§]); Occupational
Health Nurse Case Manager **(COHN/CM[§]);**
(COHN-S/CM[§]); Occupational Health Safety
Manager **(COHN/SM); (COHN-S/SM)**

ONCOLOGY NURSING
Oncology Nursing Certification Corporation[§]
125 Enterprise Dr. Pittsburgh, PA 15275-1214
oncc@ons.org
www.oncc.org

Credentials: (OCN); (AOCN); (AOCNP); (AOCNS)

OPHTHALMIC NURSING
National Certifying Board for Ophthalmic
  Registered Nurses
P.O. Box 193030
San Francisco, CA 94119
asorn@aao.org
www.asorn.org

Credential: (CRNO)

ORTHOPAEDIC NURSING
Orthopaedic Nurses Certification Board
P.O. Box 87 Columbia, SC 29202
oncb@oncb.org
www.oncb.org

Credentials: (ONC); (OCNS-C); (ONP-C)

OTORHINOLARYNGOLOGY AND
HEAD–NECK NURSES
The National Certifying Board of
  Otorhinolaryngologyand Head-Neck Nurses
202 Julia St. New Smyrna Beach, FL 32168
info@sohnnurse.com
www.sohnnurse.com

Credential: (CORLN)

PAIN MANAGEMENT[II]
American Academy of Pain Management
13947 Mono Way #A Sonora, CA 95370
aapm@aapainmanage.org
www.aapainmanage.org

Credential: (FAAPM)

PEDIATRIC NURSING[II]
Pediatric Nursing Certification Board (PNCB)
800 S. Frederick Ave., Suite 204
Gaithersburg, MD 20877-4151
info@pncb.org
www.pncb.org

Credentials: Pediatric Nurse **(CPN);** Pediatric
Nurse Practitioner **(CPNP–Primary Care); (CPNP–**
Acute Care)

PEDIATRIC ONCOLOGY
Oncology Nursing Certification Corporation
125 Enterprise Dr. Pittsburgh, PA 15275-1214
oncc@ons.org
www.oncc.org

Credential: (CPON[§])

PERIANESTHESIA NURSING
American Board of Perianesthesia Nursing
  Certification, Inc. (ABPANC)
475 Riverside Dr., 6th Floor
New York, NY 10115-0089
abpanc@proexam.org
www.cpancapa.org

Credentials: Certified Post Anesthesia Nurse
(CPAN); Certified Ambulatory Perianesthesia Nurse
(CAPA)

PERIOPERATIVE NURSING
Competency & Credentialing Institute
2170 South Parker Rd., Suite 295
Denver, CO 80231-5710
www.cc-institute.org

Credentials: (CNOR); RN First Assistant **(CRNFA)**

PLASTIC AND RECONSTRUCTIVE SURGICAL
NURSING
Plastic Surgical Nursing Certification
7794 Grow Drive Pensacola, FL 32514
aspsn@puetzamc.com
www.aspsn.org

Credential: (CPSN)

REHABILITATION NURSING
Rehabilitation Nursing Certification Board[§]
4700 W. Lake Ave. Glenview, IL 60025-1485
cert@rehabnurse.org
www.rehabnurse.org

Credential: (CRRN)

SCHOOL NURSING
National Board for Certification of
  School Nurses (NBCSN)
c/o National Association of School Nurses
1350 Broadway, Suite 1705
New York, NY 10018 (888) 776-2481
certification@nbcsn.com
www.nbcsn.com

Credential: (NCSN)

**SEXUAL ASSAULT NURSE EXAMINER—
ADULT/ADOLESCENT**
Forensic Nursing Certification Board
East Holly Ave., Box 56
Pitman, NJ 08071-0056
iafn@ajj.com
www.forensicnurse.org

Credential: (SANE-A)

UROLOGY NURSING
Certification Board for Urologic Nurses and
  Associates (CBUNA)
East Holly Ave., Box 56 Pitman, NJ 08071-0056
cbuna@ajj.com
www.suna.org

Credentials: (CURN); (CUA); (CUNP); (CUCNS); (CUPA)

WOMEN'S HEALTH/PRIMARY CARE NURSING
National Certification Corporation for the
  Obstetric, Gynecological, and Neonatal
  Nursing Specialties
P.O. Box 11082 Chicago, IL 60611-0082
www.nccnet.org

Credentials: Breastfeeding **(BF)**; Electronic Fetal
Monitoring **(EFM)**; Gynecology/Reproductive Health
Care for the Primary Care Nurse Practitioner and
Nurse Midwife **(GR)**; Inpatient Obstetric Nurse
(RNC, INPT) Low-Risk Neonatal Nurse **(RNC
and LRN)**; Maternal Newborn Nurse **(RNC, MN)**;
Menopause Clinician **(MC)** Menopause Educator
(RNC, ME) Neonatal Intensive Care Nurse **(RNC
and NIC)**; Neonatal Nurse Practitioner **(RNC)**;
Telephone Nursing Practice **(RNC, TNP)**; Women's
Health Care Nurse Practitioner **(RNC)**

WOUND, OSTOMY, AND CONTINENCE NURSING
Wound, Ostomy, and ContinenceNursing
  Certification Board
555 E. Wells St., Suite 1100
Milwaukee, WI 53202 (414)289-8721
info@wocncb.org
www.wocncb.org

Credentials: Certified Wound Ostomy Continence
Nurse **(CWOCN)**; Certified Wound Ostomy Nurse
(CWON); Certified Wound Care Nurse **(CWCN)**;
Certified Ostomy Care Nurse (COCN); Certified
Continence Care Nurse **(CCCN)**; Certified Foot Care
Nurses **(CFCN)** [†]

Source: "Your Guide to Certification," *American Journal of Nursing,* January 1, 2008, Vol.
108, Issue 1. New York, NY: Wolters Kluwer Health. Reprinted with permission.

APPENDIX B: TABLES REGARDING SALARY, EMPLOYMENT, AND OTHER DATA

TABLE 1 Demographic and Education Profiles of Registered Nurses

DEMOGRAPHIC AND EDUCATION PROFILES	TOTAL ESTIMATED PERCENT
Gender	
Male	6.6
Female	93.4
Race/ethnicity	
White	83.2
Black/African American	5.4
Asian	5.5
Native Hawaiian/Pacific Islander	0.3
American Indian/Alaskan Native	0.3
Hispanic/Latino	3.6
Age group	
<25	2.6
25–34	16
35–44	21.8
45–54	30.6
55–64	21.1
Above 65	7.5
Highest nursing or nursing-related education	
Diploma	13.9
Associate degree	36
Bachelor's	34.9
Bachelor's in related field	1.9
Master's	9.5
Master's in related field	2.8
Doctorate in nursing	0.4
Doctorate in related field	0.5

TABLE 2 Work-Related Information

WORK-RELATED INFORMATION	TOTAL ESTIMATED PERCENT
Primary employment setting	
Hospital	61.7
Nursing home/extended care facility	5.2
Academic education program	3.8
Home health setting	6.4
Community/public health setting	3.7
School health service	3.3
Occupational health	0.7
Ambulatory care setting (not hospital)	10.4
Insurance/benefits/utilization review	1.9
Other	2
Not known	0.9
Primary job title	
Staff nurse	65.9
Management/administration	12.4
Certified Registered Nurse Anesthetist	1.1
Clinical nurse specialist	0.8
Nurse midwife	0.2
Nurse practitioner	3.8
Instruction	3.7
Patient coordinator	5.4
Informatics nurse	0.9
Researcher	0.7
Surveyor/auditor/regulator	0.4
Other	2.9
Not known	0.6

TABLE 3 National Certifications for Registered Nurses

TYPES OF CERTIFICATIONS	TOTAL ESTIMATED PERCENT
Total percent of RNs who are certified	35.7
Administrator	0.3
Ambulatory	0.2
Anesthesiology	0.2
Cardiac rehabilitation	0.1
Case management	1
Community health	0.2
Critical care	1.9
Diabetes educator	0.3
Family practice	0.2
Gastroenterology	0.2
General practice	0.1
General surgery	0.9
Gerontology	0.3
Hospice/palliative care/home health	0.5
Infection control	0.1

Continued

TABLE 3 (*Continued*)

TYPES OF CERTIFICATIONS	TOTAL ESTIMATED PERCENT
Infusion therapy	0.2
Lactation consult	0.3
Legal nurse	0.2
Life support/resuscitation (BLS, ACLS, etc.)	31.2
Maternal/neonate	1.4
Medical/surgical	0.9
Neonatal intensive care	0.2
Nephrology	0.2
Neuroscience	0.2
Occupational health	0.2
Oncology	1.2
Orthopedic	0.2
Pediatrics	0.4
Psychiatric/mental health/counselor	0.6
Quality care	0.1
Registered nurse first assistant	0.1
Rehabilitation	0.4
Research	0.1
School nurse/college health	0.2
Trauma nursing/emergency medicine	4.1
Women's health	0.1
Wound care	0.2
Other	1.2

TABLE 4 Certifications in Advance Practice Registered Nursing

TYPES OF CERTIFICATIONS	TOTAL ESTIMATED PERCENT
Acute care/critical care	2.6
Adult	10.6
Anesthesia	10.6
Family	20.4
Gerontological	1.9
Midwifery	3.7
Neonatal	1.4
Pediatric	5.3
Psychiatric/mental health	4.4
Women's health care	5.2
Other	2.8

TABLE 5 Average Annual Earnings

JOB TITLE	OVERALL AVERAGE (DOLLARS)
Staff nurse	66,973
Management/administration	78,356
Certified Registered Nurse Anesthetist	154,221
Clinical nurse specialist	72,856
Nurse midwife	82,111
Nurse practitioner	85,025
Patient educator	59,491
Instruction	65,844
Patient coordinator	62,978
Informatics nurse	75,242
Consultant	76,473
Researcher	67,491
Surveyor/auditor/regulator	65,009
Other	64,003

GLOSSARY OF ACRONYMS

ACLS	Advanced Cardiac Life Support
AD	Associate Degree
AHNCC	The American Holistic Nurses' Certification Corporation
APRN	Advanced Practice Registered Nurse
BLS	Basic Life Support
BSN	Bachelors of Science in Nursing
CCRN	Critical Care Registered Nurse
CPHQ	Certified Professional Healthcare Quality
CPT	Current Procedural Terminology
DRG	Diagnostic Related Group
ECG	Electrocardiogram
ED	Emergency Department
EMT	Emergency Medical Technician
ER	Emergency Room
FDA	Food and Drug Administration
FERPA	Family Educational Rights and Privacy Act
FNP	Family Nurse Practitioner
GNP	Geriatric Nurse Practitioner
HIPPA	Health Insurance Portability and Accountability Act
IBCLC	International Board Certified Lactation Consultant
IBLCE	International Board of Lactation Consultant Examiners
ICD	International Classification of Diseases
IRB	Institutional Regulatory Board
LNC	Legal Nurse Consultant
LPN	Licensed Practical Nurse
MI	Myocardial Infarction
MSN	Masters of Science in Nursing
MPH	Masters in Public Health
NALS	Neonatal Advance Life Support
NP	Nurse Practitioner
OCN	Oncology Certified Nurse
OSHA	Occupational Safety & Health Administration
PALS	Pediatric Advance Life Support
PNP	Pediatric Nurse Practitioner

Glossary of Acronyms

PRI	Patient Review Instrument
RCIS	Registered Cardiovascular Invasive Specialist
RHIT	Registered Health Information Technician
RN	Registered Nurse
RNFA	Registered Nurse First Assist
RRA	Record Review Auditor
SANE	Sexual Assault Nurse Examiner
SNF	Skilled Nursing Facilities
TB	Tuberculosis
UAP	Unlicensed Assistive Personnel
WOCN	Wound Ostomy and Continence Nursing

■ INDEX

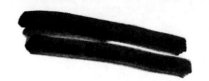

201 Careers in Nursing

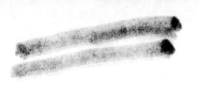